ETHICS FOR
MASSAGE THERAPISTS

ETHICS FOR MASSAGE THERAPISTS

■ TERRIE YARDLEY-NOHR, LMT

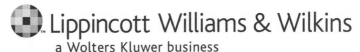
Lippincott Williams & Wilkins
a Wolters Kluwer business

Philadelphia · Baltimore · New York · London
Buenos Aires · Hong Kong · Sydney · Tokyo

Acquisitions Editor: John Goucher
Development Editors: David R. Payne, Tom Lochhaas
Marketing Manager: Hilary Henderson
Production Editor: Jennifer D.W. Glazer
Designer: Terry Mallon
Compositor: International Typesetting and Composition
Printer: RR Donnelley—Shenzhen

351 West Camden Street
Baltimore, MD 21201

530 Walnut Street
Philadelphia, PA 19106

The publisher is not responsible (as a matter of product liability, negligence, or otherwise) for any injury resulting from any material contained herein. This publication contains information relating to general principles of medical care that should not be construed as specific instructions for individual patients. Manufacturers' product information and package inserts should be reviewed for current information, including contraindications, dosages, and precautions.

Printed in China

Library of Congress Cataloging-in-Publication Data

Yardley-Nohr, Terrie.
  Ethics for massage therapists / Terrie Yardley-Nohr.
    p. ; cm.
  Includes index.
  ISBN-13: 978-0-7817-5339-5
  ISBN-10: 0-7817-5339-2
  1. Massage therapy—Moral and ethical aspects. I. Title.
  [DNLM: 1. Massage—ethics. 2. Codes of Ethics. 3. Professional-Patient Relations—ethics. WB 537 Y27e 2007]
  RM721.Y37 2007
  615.8'22—dc22   2006013739

The publishers have made every effort to trace the copyright holders for borrowed material. If they have inadvertently overlooked any, they will be pleased to make the necessary arrangements at the first opportunity.

To purchase additional copies of this book, call our customer service department at **(800) 638-3030** or fax orders to **(301) 223-2320.** International customers should call **(301) 223-2300.**

Visit Lippincott Williams & Wilkins on the Internet: http://www.LWW.com. Lippincott Williams & Wilkins customer service representatives are available from 8:30 am to 6:00 pm, EST.

12
6 7 8 9 10 11

RRS1206

Dedicated to massage students now entering the massage profession and to the many practicing massage therapists who have laid an ethical foundation for them to follow.

PREFACE

When entering the field of massage therapy, students rarely think about ethics and the profound effect ethics can have on their career. Students are always taught the technical skills needed to become good bodyworkers, but often too little time is spent teaching and discussing ethics, students' own personal beliefs, and the beliefs clients bring to their massage therapy sessions. Often a new therapist is surprised by clients' questions or concerns and are at a loss for how to address situations that commonly arise.

In massage therapy classes, students seem continually to raise questions about how to handle many situations they will encounter in practice. Often these have little to do with the technical skills of massage therapy but rather involve values, morals, and ethical questions. Unsure what to do, some students may try to take a hard line with clients or not address an issue at all. Neither approach is a good solution for the client or therapist, however, and neither contributes to a healthy therapeutic relationship. The alternative is to study ethical principles and think about issues one will face in practice, and thereby become prepared to prevent most problems and comfortably manage situations when they do arise.

This book originated in a commitment to help massage students begin their new career with a firm foundation: knowing who they are and what they believe and why. Building on this foundation, students will be able to learn to accept the wide variety and diversity of clients, many with very different backgrounds, whom they will encounter in practice. Balancing the art and science of massage therapy with ethical behavior and good interpersonal skills takes practice, but all students can be successful when they are prepared to do so.

This text begins with an exploration of self and gradually builds to a larger understanding of clients' needs and expectations. Many resources within the profession of massage therapy can help students begin their career, and this text frequently encourages the use of such resources. Building from the material presented here, students and new practitioners of massage therapy can then develop their own code of ethics to ensure a safe and effective environment for both them and their clients.

PEDAGOGICAL FEATURES

To aid in learning, the following pedagogical features have been included in this text:

- **Chapter preview:** a chapter-opening bulleted list briefly introducing key chapter topics.
- **Key terms:** special terms that students should learn will be boldfaced at their first use in the chapter, listed and defined at the beginning of the chapter, and included in the glossary at the back of the book.
- **Key point boxes:** boxes appearing occasionally throughout each chapter that summarize key points in bulleted lists.
- **Exercises:** various review and thought-provoking exercises sprinkled throughout each chapter that students can complete on their own to help learn and review the chapter content.
- **Scenarios:** realistic massage therapy scenarios with critical thinking questions that prompt the student to apply the knowledge they have learned in the chapter.
- **Case studies:** extended case examples of massage therapists and their clients that illustrate ethical concepts discussed in the chapter.
- **Code of ethics:** sample codes of ethics.
- **Personal journal:** write-in exercises in which students explore their own thoughts and feelings, such as inventorying their attitudes, exploring past events that relate to how they feel now about touch, etc.
- **Chapter summary:** brief paragraph at chapter's end to pull it all back together.
- **Additional activities:** end-of-chapter review and learning activities that are in addition to the exercises appearing sporadically throughout each chapter.

User's Guide

Ethics for Massage Therapists provides you with a structured format for learning ethics in the field of massage therapy. In the book, you will find a discussion of core industry standards of practice, laws, morals, rules, and regulations for building an ethical practice.

Look for these learning features inside:

CHAPTER PREVIEW & KEY TERMS

Orient you to the information presented in the chapter. ▶

> ### CHAPTER PREVIEW
>
> ■ Disclosure as sharing information with other health care providers or your clients
>
> ■ Client disclosure of information about their health history for the safe practice of massage
>
> ■ Nondisclosure of information placing the client at risk during massage
>
> ■ Third-party disclosure as a health care provider sharing information with another party
>
> ■ HIPAA regulations guaranteeing the information rights and responsibilities of patients and health care providers
>
> ■ Therapist disclosure of information regarding treatment, outcomes, credentials, and personal health issues to clients
>
> ■ Ethical behavior involving knowing the boundaries related to disclosure
>
> ### KEY TERMS
>
> **Beliefs:** what you personally feel is true
>
> **Culture:** the customary beliefs, habits, and traits of a racial, religious, or social group, often depending on one's country and language
>
> **Ethics:** an individual's or group's standards of behavior
>
> **Morals:** beliefs about what is right and wrong or good and bad
>
> **Values:** something of worth or held in esteem

> **BOX 8-1** | *Helpful Hints to Ensure Client Disclosure*
>
> 1. Include a brief paragraph on your health history form explaining the reasons for asking about clients' health.
> 2. Look for clues in the client's answers on the health history form, such as fever, fatigue, soreness, etc.
> 3. When in doubt, ask the client questions during the oral interview.
> 4. Watch for signs and symptoms that could mean the client has a condition that could contraindicate massage.
> 5. Keep good notes and records of your session with clients. You may see patterns develop that need further investigation.
> 6. Ask clients at the beginning of each session for any new information about their health.
> 7. Include on your form a statement that the client has disclosed all known health information. The client should sign and date this statement. This helps prevent clients from knowingly not disclosing health information, and helps protect you legally if the client has not disclosed a condition that could become worse with massage.
> 8. Always be honest in recording information that you have learned. Clients have no argument with a professional who is honest.

◀ **BOXES**

Break down important information into an easy to understand format.

YOUR PERSONAL JOURNALS

Require you to reflect on important ethical issues and ask important questions regarding those issues. ▶

> ### Your Personal Journal
>
> This chapter has frequently asked you to think about your life and how you have come to believe and feel as you now do. Take a few minutes now to reflect on your thoughts and feelings about bodywork and why you have chosen this profession (Fig. 1-2).
>
> Be as honest with yourself as you can—these are not thoughts you need to share with anyone else.
>
> 1. What is your general view of bodywork?
>
> 2. Why do you feel it is a valuable career?
>
> 3. What is your biggest fear?

EXERCISE 5-3

Practicing how to talk to a client who makes an inappropriate request should be an important part of your training.

Pair up with another student. One is the therapist and the other the client. Use props as needed (desk and chair, massage table, massage chair). Different pairs of students use the following scenarios. Take the time to compose your scenario and present it to the class. Afterwards, the rest of the class should offer suggestions for how to handle the incident.

1. A new client calls to make an appointment for a massage. He asks a lot of questions including what the therapist will be wearing.

2. A female client tells her male therapist that she would like to have lunch with him sometime soon.

3. A male client asks his female therapist for advice about a problem in his marriage. He keeps bringing it up during the session.

4. A male client does not like to be draped and keeps taking the draping off during the session.

EXERCISES

Questions throughout the chapter require you to reflect on the information learned and form opinions about ethical & unethical behavior. ▶

SCENARIO

Samuel had been practicing massage for 5 years at a very busy resort spa. In this time he built up a regular clientele who often requested him for their vacation massages. Two week ago, Samuel learned from his doctor that he was HIV-positive. Although personally devastated by the news, he was not worried about his massage practice. The doctor reassured him that he would likely not develop AIDS for many years to come and could possibly lead a very normal life for a decade or more. The doctor also gave him information about how HIV is spread and precautions to take. Samuel read all of the information. He knew that HIV is not spread through skin-to-skin contact but understood that he must watch carefully for any breaks in his skin or other ways his body fluids might infect others. Samuel now must decide if he will tell his employers and his clients.

Discuss the following questions, considering each possible action:

1. Should Samuel tell his employers and clients? What are the advantages and disadvantages of telling and not telling?
2. Is there one ethically and professionally correct thing to do?
3. List possible ways Samuel could handle this situation while being ethical and professional.

◀ SCENARIOS & SCENARIO QUESTIONS

Present you with practice-based scenarios so that you are able to apply information learned in the text to a working environment. Questions at the end of each scenario require you to think critically about the situation at hand.

CASE STUDIES

Practice-based situations where the massage practitioner faces an ethical issue. ▶

CASE STUDY

A female bodyworker has had regular sessions with a male client for about 6 months when he begins to ask her personal questions. He asks if she has a boyfriend and says he'd like to take her out sometime. She tries to avoid his questions as best she can and tries to change the subject and continue with the session. Over the next few sessions, however, he continues to ask more about her personal life. It is getting hard for her to avoid this conversation. He finally asks if she would like to have dinner with him soon. She tells the client that it is against her profession's code of ethics to become personally involved with a client and that she will not go out with him as long as he is a client. This answer lets the client know that the professional code encompasses what she as a therapist can and cannot do.

KEY POINTS

Summarize essential information in bulleted lists throughout each chapter. ▶

Key Points

- It is important to know both parties' expectations.
- Expectations can frequently change.
- Group dynamics play an important role in conflicts and resolution.
- Policies and procedures can help prevent conflicts.
- Conflicts between a therapist and client can be prevented with good communication.

ADDITIONAL ACTIVITIES

After you and your classmates have a sense of what laws and rules apply to a massage therapy practice in your area, have a class discussion to answer these questions:

1. What areas of the law or rules protect clients?
2. What areas of the law protect therapists?
3. Do any areas of law restrict the practice of massage or cause hardship for therapists?
4. Do any areas of law need more definition?
5. How many of the therapists you and your classmates interviewed were well educated about laws and regulations?
6. How would you go about changing a law or rule that needs revision?

◀ ADDITIONAL ACTIVITIES

At the end of each chapter, these activities require you to seek out more information on the topics covered in the chapter and apply the ethical issues covered in a practical way.

REVIEWERS

Rachelle Ackerman, CMT
Instructor
Community College of Vermont
Brattleboro, Vermont

Naomi Heivilin
Synergy Massage
Madison, Wisconsin

Judith Klein, BA, LMT
Instructor, Clinical Director
Sarasota School of Massage Therapy
Sarasota, Florida

Cheryl L. Siniakin, PhD
Director, Massage Therapy Program
Community College of Allegheny County, Allegheny Campus
Pittsburgh, Pennsylvania

Michael Sullivan, BS
Assistant Professor, Program Coordinator
Anne Arundel Community College
Arnold, Maryland

ACKNOWLEDGMENTS

I first thank some very special people at Lippincott Williams & Wilkins. Pete Darcy, thank you for asking me to write this book. You saw something in a conversation that we had that made you think that I could do this. Tom Lochhaas, you are truly an artist. You have helped me find the words to express my ideas. Thank you from the bottom of my heart—I could not have done this without you. David Payne, thank you for your patience and your guidance. You made it look easy during the challenging times. Thanks also to the staff of Lippincott Williams & Wilkins. You are truly a remarkable team as well as a great asset and resource for the massage therapy profession.

Thank you to Brenda Griffith, Fred Engel, Cheryl Siniakin, Elliot Greene, Chris Voltarel, and Carolyn Talley-Porter for your contributions, and to my many friends in the American Massage Therapy Association (AMTA) for your support.

Thanks also to all the therapists who took part in the peer review of the manuscript drafts of this book. Your feedback was immeasurable and helped expand on many sections of this book.

To my family and friends—thank you for being patient and understanding all the times I needed to be at my computer. Jenni, Chris, and Drea—I hope you are proud of what is written here. To my Mom: when I sat and watched you read my first chapter, you warmed my heart. To my Dad: I know you are watching over me from above. You instilled in me much of what is in this book.

This book is written for every student I have had the privilege of teaching. Each student has brought me new questions, concerns, and approaches to situations that arise in the field of massage therapy. I have seen your fears and concerns, and I truly hope that this book will help you address the many issues that affect all new therapists in their massage career.

CONTENTS

YOUR BELIEF SYSTEM

KEY TERMS

Beliefs: what you personally feel is true

Culture: the customary beliefs, habits, and traits of a racial, religious, or social group, often depending on one's country and language

Ethics: an individual's or group's standards of behavior

Morals: beliefs about what is right and wrong or good and bad

Values: something of worth or held in esteem

Our society is composed of people with many different belief systems and cultural backgrounds. Different individuals and groups have distinctly different **beliefs** about what they consider wrong or right. For example, capital punishment is viewed as acceptable by some people and some cultures and not by others. Different personal histories also influence what different people believe and follow in their everyday lives. Within the same culture, for example, individuals often view issues very differently. Are such issues as the appropriate age for dating or premarital sex personal choices or are they moral issues? Different people see these issues in different ways. Personal beliefs also involve simple, day-to-day issues such as following rules at work, etiquette, and even things that some people believe are common sense. Many, many factors play a part in how these different beliefs came about.

As an individual, you have your own belief system that influences you every day, often moment by moment, without you even realizing it is affecting how you think, talk, and act. When driving, for example, you know that it is against the law to make a U turn in the middle of an intersection, so most of the time you naturally make your turn somewhere else without giving it a second thought. You believe that following the law is the right thing to do. When you see someone else making an illegal turn, you may believe that person is breaking the law. This is just one simple example of how our beliefs affect our daily actions.

In this chapter you will explore your personal belief system and consider how it formed. Understanding your own personal beliefs and values is important in the profession of massage and bodywork, because these beliefs and values contribute to your personal ethical principles. Examining the varied aspects of your personal beliefs, values, morals, and ethics will help you develop guidelines for your successful practice in bodywork. Success in the practice in bodywork means not only financial success but also, first and foremost, development of valuable and healthy therapeutic relationships with your clients and peers. A solid foundation for your practice helps reassure both clients and other therapists.

In this chapter and the ones that follow, we discuss how to increase your understanding of your own values and ethics, examining where you are now and looking ahead to what is needed in your practice.

Key Points

- Understanding your personal beliefs is important.
- Beliefs and morals are learned.
- Your beliefs contribute to a successful massage therapy practice.

PERSONAL DEVELOPMENT OF VALUES

FAMILY INFLUENCES

Often when individuals are asked who had the greatest influence on their lives, they naturally answer their parents or other close family members, relatives, or friends. This is understandable because it is these individuals with whom you spend most of your time during your first 15 to 18 years. Your family members likely were your caretakers and provided the essentials you needed. Their influence on your belief system starts as soon as you are born and often continues even after you leave home. After adolescence, other valued people will have influence, such as teachers, a spouse, close friends, and even your own children.

As a toddler, you begin learning right and wrong by being told so by other people. Your mother or caretaker tells you not to hit your sister or pull the dog's tail. You are told to look both ways before crossing the street and that it's not nice to make fun of people. Children generally trust what others tell them and often develop conditioned responses to many situations. After you begin school, other people begin to influence what you consider right and wrong. Teachers and other influences may reinforce what you have learned or may present a different point of view. When receiving conflicting points of view, individuals may eventually reformulate what they believe is right or wrong, or may hold to their original beliefs.

As you enter the adolescent years, still more influences are introduced. Information and influences extend beyond the smaller world of family and school and begin to involve the larger world. Peers have a great influence on what you value and how you think and act. Television, radio, and the Internet provide a large amount of information and have been shown to influence people's belief systems. Because individuals today have much information readily available and are exposed to a huge amount of diverse and different information, it is easy to understand that many people question their learned values, even at an early age. Available information includes diverse information about other societies, beliefs, religions, and cultures. With so many influences, which can often be conflicting, it is not unusual that many teens rebel against what they have learned within their family. Adolescents are exposed to many different viewpoints in school and various social settings and may begin to look elsewhere for a broader understanding of what is right and wrong.

Up until adolescence, most individuals have listened to what their caretakers say about things that happen in the world. You may have adopted your family's values and beliefs about many things, including ideas as simple as thinking a mother should stay at home to raise children to more complex beliefs such as religious beliefs. You may have heard your caretakers or other adults, for example, make positive or negative comments about other cultures and their beliefs. This could have a profound effect on how you respond when you meet a person from another country.

When family members feel that something is wrong, they typically express their unhappiness or anger about it. Because you are raised this way and frequently hear such comments, you too may believe the same thing or have the same feelings. This is only natural because what family members say is very important to you. It may not be until you are older and have been exposed to other points of view and information that you begin to see things in a different light.

When you leave your family and are living on your own, you likely have a new sense of freedom. Without even realizing it you may continue to rely on your previous beliefs, or you may develop new beliefs and values. Living on your own can test what you think to be wrong or right. It is natural for a person to try new ways of doing things. It is a way to test the old ideas and look for something new. Many lessons are learned and sometimes, as the old saying goes, "You have to learn the hard way." Making a mistake often causes a shift in your thinking and leads to evaluating what you may do differently in the future.

In adulthood, however, most people's values and beliefs are fairly well formulated. Often individuals end up still believing in some of the values that were instilled in them in their youth, although some differences may have developed as a result of their own life experiences. At the same time, as an adult, you are interacting with a wider range of people in the world and may experience conflicts between your values and beliefs and those of other individuals (Fig. 1-1).

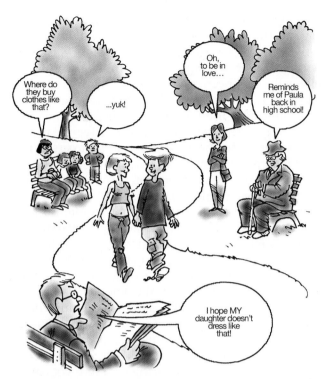

FIGURE 1-1 ■ Because of differences in background and many other factors, people have a wide variety of values and beliefs.

As you form a serious relationship with another person, for example, a common source of conflict is differences in what you feel is right and wrong. Conflicts can occur over things as simple as a difference in opinion about doing housework or preparing meals. Larger conflicts in belief systems may involve religion, cultural customs, or family customs. Mature adults, however, can learn to compromise and be flexible while respecting the different beliefs of others—although if two parties have strong opposing beliefs, a conflict could occur. As you will see later in this chapter and in Chapter 2, some values may involve serious ethical or moral beliefs, and then you will need to decide whether or not you should compromise.

> *Key Points*
> ■ We learn through developmental stages.
> ■ Family influences are important.
> ■ Beliefs vary from person to person.

Thinking about your past will help you see how you have come to believe what you do today. The influences of three people in your life involve just a tiny fraction of all the influences on your beliefs to this point in your life. In the following sections, you will see how other factors also have influenced your present values.

EXERCISE 1-1

Think about three people you believe have influenced you. Try to name at least one value or belief that each person helped instill in you. Remember that beliefs and values can be either a positive value or a negative value (for or against something). Finally, reflect on whether you think this belief or value helps you or hinders you in today's society.

Person belief or value	Affects you how today?

INFLUENCES OF CULTURE

The culture in which you were raised has a lot to do with how you think and believe. **Culture** can be defined as the customary beliefs, habits, and traits of a racial, religious, or social group, often depending on one's country and language. Therefore you can think of culture as the larger environment surrounding a group of people. America is one culture, but within most cultures there are many subcultures involving different ethnic origins, religions, geographical features, and belief systems. Steeped within cultures and subcultures are many traditions, such as holidays, clothing, and food preferences. Staying close to the environment in which they were raised often gives individuals a safe feeling.

The term "culture shock" refers to the experience of suddenly encountering a very different environment outside one's familiar culture. For some, this causes stress. For others, exposure to other cultures leads to reconsideration of their own values and more respect for the diversity of thoughts and traditions of other cultures. Think about the environment that you were raised in and what you have learned from it. Think about the times you may have gone to stay with a friend and how different that friend's family traditions and environment may have been. Which of your values or beliefs might have been very different if you had grown up in a different culture?

INFLUENCES OF ENVIRONMENT

Physical environmental factors also influence how you think and what you believe. If you were raised on a farm and moved into the city when you went to college, you might initially have a hard time adjusting to crowds and the hustle and bustle and noises of the city. Likewise, if you grew up in a large city and then moved to a small town, you may have trouble adjusting to the quiet and relaxed environment of many small towns. Yet, in either situation, adapting to a new environment can help you both better understand ways of living and help broaden your values and beliefs.

The environment includes not only the physical surroundings but also the people who inhabit an area. Particular groups or populations often possess particular beliefs and habits. A community's shared beliefs are generally influenced by traditions and the community's success in coping with its traditions, habits, and beliefs. Beliefs and values can be very different in different places. A massage therapist opening a practice in one town may be looked upon as a welcome addition to the community, while in a different community another therapist may encounter opposition due to ordinances or rules enacted in the past to drive out prostitution.

Why are these two environments so different? One community may have had problems with prostitution at some point in the past and now associates massage with prostitution. Many illegal businesses have in the past advertised using the term "massage." In addition, change can be threatening to a community's sense of comfort if people like the way things have always been. Furthermore, a profession like massage therapy that involves touching a person's body often threatens some individuals' comfort zone. In large part this attitude results from misinformation and misunderstandings about what massage and bodywork professionals truly do. Later chapters discuss working with the public and educating others about your new profession.

Key Points

- Beliefs gradually become values.
- Values are part of who you are.
- Understanding our past help us understand our present.
- We are influenced by culture, environment, and the world at large.

EXPOSURE TO THE WORLD

The exposure you have had to world events, news, education, and other cultures and belief systems also greatly influences how you think. The thought processes of people who have lived most of their lives sheltered from other ways of thinking and doing things generally reflect only what they know and have seen themselves. Their beliefs and values may be more directly attributed to their upbringing in the family and immediate environment. This is not to say that their beliefs are in any way wrong or not as important as those of someone else who has been more broadly exposed to the world. It is true, however, that there are many ways of seeing and interpreting information, and the more exposure a person has to outside ideas and information, the more information that person has on which to base beliefs and values.

Modes of communication, especially, have changed dramatically in the last decade, as have people's exposure to information communicated through the media. A few decades ago, newspapers were the main source of information, often providing a great deal of information about events. As television became the main source of news for a large segment of the population, the amount of coverage about individual events on the evening news decreased to a small fraction of the information presented in newspapers. People watching television often received a thumbnail sketch of the news, while those reading newspapers often got more detail. Now many people receive their information primarily from the Internet, which allows them to pick out only what they want to learn on any given topic. At the same time, however, many people are concerned that some of this information may be inaccurate or biased, and that many individuals may not be receiving the larger picture. Nonetheless, all of these sources of information continue to influence our beliefs and values.

On the positive side, many people today have more information available on which to formulate their opinions and beliefs. The media has played an important role in helping people see the benefits of massage. Only a few years ago, the only mentions of massage in the news generally involved stories about a massage parlor or some illicit activity. Today, hundreds of news stories, articles, and Internet sites explain the different massage modalities and their positive effects. For example, news readers or viewers may see a story about the positive effects of massage for premature babies in a hospital. Exposure to the outside world can influence us in many different ways. These factors are another dimension to consider as you analyze your present beliefs and values and try to sort out what things in your past have led you to become the person you are today.

VALUES TO BELIEFS

When does a belief become a valued part of your life? This is an important question when evaluating

EXERCISE 1-2

Think about how your beliefs and values have come about. Answering the questions below will help you realize the sources of your present beliefs.

1. Name two people who were strong influences for you as a child.

2. Can you remember a phrase or saying from each of these people that sticks in your mind?

3. During your adolescence, do you remember any values or beliefs of your caretakers that you questioned?

4. What led to you questioning these values or beliefs?

5. What resulted from your questioning? Did your belief change?

what is important in our belief and value systems. If you were to count how many times a day you say or think, "I believe that ...," you may be surprised. We say things like this frequently when we believe that something is true or right. If you say, "I believe the store is two blocks down the street on the right," you are saying you *think* this is true but you are open to the possibility that it is not precisely true. But if you say, "The store is two block down the street on the right," you are saying you *know* this is true. See the difference? The second statement is, for you, an absolute statement of fact, that it *is* where you say it is.

The same holds true for many beliefs and values. When you believe in something, when you really feel its importance, you know it is the right thing to believe or do. When that belief becomes part of your value system, you take ownership and it becomes part of who and what you are. When you *know* something is right or wrong, and you see no room for exceptions, this belief has become a valued part of who you are. Think about this when you are speaking to others, and notice when you say "I know" versus "I believe."

Something that you value is a strong part of your foundation. For example, saying "I believe I will not take financial advantage of a client" does not mean quite the same thing as "I will never take financial advantage of a client." The process by which beliefs

and values become your foundation is important for becoming an ethical person.

VALUES AND MORALS

When does a value become a moral belief? Remember, a **value** is anything you hold to be important, while a **moral** is a strong belief that something is always right or wrong. You may value personal hygiene, for example, but it is unlikely you would consider it immoral not to brush your teeth first thing in the morning. Other values do become morals, however. You may believe it is immoral to steal or to harm another person. These are personal values about serious matters of right and wrong. Often people think of morals as absolutes, such as saying it is never moral for anyone in any place at any time to steal from another. For many people, morality is based on religious beliefs. As well, a country's laws are usually based on a shared moral system about what is right and wrong. For example, the law against murder reflects the shared moral belief that murder is wrong.

Ethical beliefs are similar to moral beliefs but are not exactly the same. For many people, **ethics** depends somewhat on the situation; it is not an absolute principle. For example, you may believe that it is wrong to lie to people. Does that mean you would never, ever lie to anyone in any situation? Most of us can easily think of situations where being completely honest could hurt another person or when we might instead "tell a little white lie." Does that mean we have committed an immoral act? Most of us would likely say no, that we did the right thing because it was more important not to hurt the other person than it was to be brutally honest. We value telling the truth, and it is an ethical principle for how we live, but it is not a moral absolute. In everyday conversation people often use the words "moral" and "ethical" as if they mean the same thing, but it is sometimes important to distinguish between the two.

In the same way, we should distinguish between law and ethics. Certain business practices, for example, are illegal, and a business can be punished for breaking these laws. Other situations, however, involve ethical principles. It may be legal for a business to increase its prices when demand for an item is high, but some may question whether this is ethical. Remember: *ethics involves standards of behavior,* not simply moral issues of right and wrong or legal questions of what the law requires.

In a day-to-day massage therapy practice, we are seldom confronted with larger issues of morality or

EXERCISE 1-3

Find an article in a newspaper that identifies an ethical problem. (Ethical issues are often discussed in relation to business, politics, or even sports.) Read the article and report to the class what the situation was and how it involved an issue of ethical behavior.

_____

_____

_____

_____

_____

_____

legality. But ethical issues may often arise. How much training should I have in a certain technique before I perform it on a client? How honest should I be when a client asks me what I think about another health care professional? Is it appropriate to become close friends with one of my clients? These involve potential ethical issues. Such questions are not always easily answered—that's the reason for a book like this. You can begin to understand such issues, however, by first understanding what you value right now in your life, and then building on that foundation as you develop professional ethics for your practice.

DEFINING YOUR BELIEFS IN THE BODYWORK PROFESSION

As a student studying for a career in massage or bodywork, you may have heard comments about your new career from family members, friends, or co-workers. You may well have the support of your family and friends. Yet, students sometimes have concerns about comments that are not flattering or may even be intimidating. It is perfectly natural to feel angry or hurt by such comments. In the past, massage was linked in many people's minds with undesirable behaviors such as prostitution, and the mere mention of the word massage may make some people think you are entering an unsavory career. It is perfectly natural that some people who do not understand the profession of massage therapy may have different values or beliefs about it. Later, we discuss how to deal with such situations.

It is just as important, however, to understand your own beliefs about a career in bodywork and

massage. Developing your own code of ethics, what you value or believe is right or wrong in your profession, will help you feel at ease and be comfortable with and proud of the work you do. During your training you will learn a great deal about the effects and benefits of massage, all of which you can use when talking with someone who has a different view of the profession. Clients, other health professionals, and the general public will gain a strong respect for who you are when they understand the benefits of massage and see how your values and beliefs are part of who you are as a practitioner. Your foundation needs to encompass not only massage skills and techniques but also your beliefs and values. It is important to present to others a strong foundation so that they feel they will be treated in an effective and safe way.

Always remember that people have different values and beliefs that have been shaped by their own past life experiences, just as your values and beliefs were shaped by yours. Your own strong sense of identity will help you through situations when your own values may be in conflict with others.

COPING WITH DIFFERENT BELIEFS ABOUT MASSAGE

The general public has many different thoughts, attitudes, and beliefs about massage and bodywork. The media have helped spread the word about the positive effects of many different modalities. The growing number of massage therapists and different facilities that offer massage has increased the public's exposure to bodywork. Massage therapists often offer the public information

EXERCISE 1-4

Beside each word below, write the first word that comes to your mind.

massage _____

touch _____

masseuse _____

spa _____

boundaries _____

bodywork _____

ethics _____

Do you see a pattern in your responses? Try to describe it.

_____

Your Personal Journal

This chapter has frequently asked you to think about your life and how you have come to believe and feel as you now do. Take a few minutes now to reflect on your thoughts and feelings about bodywork and why you have chosen this profession (Fig. 1-2).

Be as honest with yourself as you can—these are not thoughts you need to share with anyone else.

1. What is your general view of bodywork?

2. Why do you feel it is a valuable career?

3. What is your biggest fear?

4. What comments from others have made you angry or hurt your feelings?

5. What do you do when these comments are made?

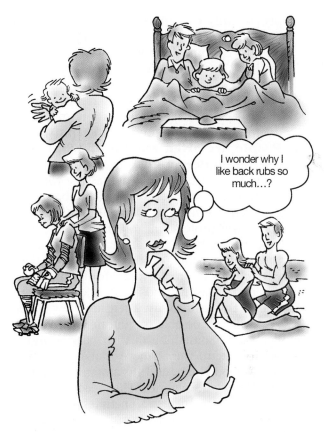

FIGURE 1-2 ■ Both ideas and emotional responses are shaped by many factors in our background.

You will learn how to turn a negative situation into a positive, educational experience. Following are some guidelines that may help you when someone makes a negative comment.

1. **Don't get angry or defensive.** You have nothing to defend. You are training in a wonderful career that has a very valuable place in society today. Instead of getting angry, take a moment to share your enthusiasm. You might begin by saying, "You may not know how many doctors these days are sending their patients to massage therapists. Lots of research has shown how massage helps people become much healthier."

2. **The person who made the comment may just be kidding.** Friends and family do like to have fun with each other. You might say, "I know a lot of people think being a massage therapist is not a real career, but I can't wait to work in the health care community and help people feel better."

3. **If a comment is truly out of line, take the opportunity to educate.** An important responsibility of all massage therapists is to educate the public about what they do. Most negative comments are made because

about massage. Chair massage in public venues has helped increase the public's awareness of massage and is the first massage experience for many.

Even with all this positive information available, at times, unfortunately, some people still make negative comments about massage that are hurtful or may make you angry. Some students of massage therapy feel they sometimes have to defend their new career to family or friends. As you continue your training, you will gain more information that can help you cope with situations like this. Over time, you will feel more comfortable talking about your career and the healthful effects of massage.

people truly do not understand this type of work. You might say, "There are so many misconceptions about what massage therapy really is. To practice in most locations, we are required to have extensive training, such as a minimum of 500 hours of school. In most states we are a licensed profession, much like doctors, nurses, and physical therapists."

4. **People are often fearful of what they do not understand.** Educating the public about the positive values of massage will help them learn what bodywork is all about. You can help calm their fears with information about the profession. You might say, "Massage therapists are educating the public about the positive benefits of massage and working with clients to provide the safe and nurturing aspects of massage and bodywork."

5. **Learn to walk away.** There are a few people you will not be able to educate or convince. Because of something in their background or belief system, they believe that bodywork is not a good thing, and no amount of talking will change their minds. These people will not become your clients. Sometimes it is better just to say nothing at all.

As you understand better how people's values and beliefs develop, you will understand more fully why others think the way they do. You will see some diversity in beliefs even within your own classroom. It is good to discuss differences and to accept this diversity. Remember: there seldom is one right way to think or one best belief. Keep an open mind about what others think and say. This can be a valuable learning tool. You will encounter a wide diversity of clients in your new profession, and it is important to be able to understand how others think.

Your values and beliefs contribute to your own personal code of ethics, which along with the professional ethics you will learn will determine how you act and treat other professionals and clients. Your values and beliefs will help you set boundaries and parameters that ensure safety for both you and your clients.

SUMMARY

Values and beliefs are a personal reflection of who you are and what you believe. As we begin to form values and beliefs in childhood, we also learn how we should behave in different situations. Eventually our values and beliefs become our personal code of action, which may be similar to or different from other people's.

Values, beliefs, ethics, and morals are all important aspects of successful businesses and professionals today. The general public and other health care professionals pay considerable attention to our professional values, beliefs, and behavior. Understanding who you are and where your values and beliefs came from is a starting point for developing professional ethics.

SCENARIO

Susan has just begun her practice as a massage therapist. Her mother is a nurse, and Susan grew up with a great respect for all the health professions and how they can make a difference in people's lives by helping them regain or maintain their health. She chose massage therapy as her profession in part because she enjoys hands-on work and in part because of her own experience with massage, which played a major role in her recovery from a serious sports injury in high school. In her massage therapy program everyone acted very professionally and accepted the value of professional massage.

Now, just a month into her practice, she has experienced some negative comments from others. At a party recently she was introduced as a masseuse, leading a couple of people to make tasteless jokes about her profession and how easy it would be to "pick up guys." Susan found it very difficult to respond to those comments.

In small groups, discuss various ways to answer these questions.

1. What are some potential ways that Susan could have responded to the comments?
2. Explain how this situation could be turned into an educational opportunity.
3. Do you feel that this type of obstacle would be challenging if you experienced it? What can you do to cope if this occurs to you?

Key Points

■ Massage has historical associations we need to understand.
■ Understanding your own beliefs about bodywork is important.
■ Professional values lead to pride in your work.
■ Learning how to cope with comments from others is important.
■ Accept diversity.

VALUES AND EMOTIONS

2

All individuals have their own beliefs, values, and morals. We may have similar beliefs about many things, but there are also significant differences among people. In the previous chapter, you saw why people's beliefs and values vary and gained a better understanding of how your own beliefs, values, and ethics developed. Because you personally own and take pride in your beliefs, you naturally are often emotional about them. In this chapter, you will learn how your values and emotions and your client's values and emotions may be the same or may conflict, how problems may develop and can be resolved, and how emotions are involved in ethics.

BELIEFS AND FEELINGS

When you strongly believe in something, it is only natural for you to believe it is true. But as we saw in Chapter 1, beliefs are not the same as facts, and two people can have two different beliefs about the same realities. In an ideal world we could all talk openly and calmly about our beliefs and understand the

difference between facts and beliefs—and then we might more easily respect the different beliefs of others. In reality, however, we are often very emotional about what we believe. This emotion makes it more difficult to recognize that other people are not necessarily wrong when they believe something else. A classic health care example is abortion: people on both sides of this issue often have very emotional beliefs about whether abortion is right or wrong. As in most issues involving beliefs, there is no simple answer—no "facts" that definitively prove either side's position. People on both sides of the issue may have the same information but perceive it differently. Many such issues are prevalent in our society today, and in most instances you can observe how strongly people *feel* about what they believe.

When our emotions are involved, we tend to take a stronger stand on what we believe. The issues become more personal, and we can be reluctant to listen to others who believe differently. This occurs frequently, for example, in political campaigns. Politicians take positions on issues they feel strongly about. Examples are human rights, universal health care, and taxes. They have strong feelings about what they believe is the right thing for our government to do. Campaigns often become very heated because of the emotions attached to these beliefs. Voters often agree or disagree with these beliefs and vote accordingly, often with just as much emotion. But again, there is usually no simple "truth" that makes positions right or wrong—these are different beliefs that result in part from different personal backgrounds and in part from different interpretations of information. A variety of interpretations can and should be expected—this is part of what makes our world so interesting and diverse. But what about the emotions associated with these different beliefs? Strong emotions can have positive effects when they motivate individuals to act as they believe but can have negative effects when they get in the way of understanding another person's beliefs and feelings.

Emotions are similarly very important in a massage therapy practice. In fact, the situation is very similar to voting for a candidate: clients who disagree with your values, beliefs, or ethics most likely would have reservations about becoming a client. A client who is not comfortable with how you act, talk, or behave may not feel comfortable working with you in a massage setting.

Clients with a wide variety of beliefs and values will enter your practice. A therapist who turned away all clients with different beliefs would have a very small practice. Learning to accept diversity and working with clients in a professional manner are part of being a successful therapist. Remember that clients take ownership of their beliefs just as you do with yours, and it is important to respect the differences.

Communication between the client and therapist during a session is important. Checking in with clients on pressure and pain levels and addressing issues pertinent to the session are important aspects of a therapeutic relationship. But some clients will start to talk about other issues or personal matters. Talkative clients may just be nervous or friendly, or they may be trying to avoid issues that come up through bodywork. Listening to a client talking about personal beliefs or other matters may start the therapist thinking about his or her own beliefs, resulting in a loss of focus on the work being done. It then is important to be aware of what is happening and redirect your focus back to the session. Often it can be difficult not to engage in conversation with the client, especially when the client is asking you questions. Bring the client back to a focus on the session through an emphasis on breathing and talking about the goal for the session. It is important not to start talking about your own feelings and beliefs during the session, especially on topics that have nothing to do with the session itself.

> *Key Points*
> - Strong emotions are often attached to beliefs.
> - Emotional reactions can harm the therapist–client relationship.
> - Professionalism helps avoid conflicts.

YOUR OWN FEELINGS

When you first began to think about doing bodywork for a living, do you remember any reservations you may have had? Consider these in Exercise 2-1.

Most massage therapy students enter school with some concerns or mixed feelings about doing bodywork for a living. For example, some students cannot imagine having to massage someone's feet. Most schools teach massage techniques for the feet, some even incorporating reflexology and the zones of the feet. Some students may hope they can get by in

---

EXERCISE 2-1

Answer the following questions regarding your feelings about the bodywork profession.

1. What initial reservations did you have about touching clients?

   _____

   _____

2. Who did you express these concerns to? (Or have you expressed these concerns to anybody?)

   _____

   _____

3. Could these reservations lead to any problems? How might these reservations affect your clients?

   _____

   _____

4. What can you do to help resolve these concerns?

   _____

   _____

Share your answers with other students or discuss these in class. You may find that other classmates share the same concerns. Finding possible solutions can help alleviate some of your fears.

their practice without working on a client's feet, but for many clients, having their feet worked on is one of the best parts of a massage. Think about your feelings for a moment: do you personally not like to have your feet worked on, or is it that you do not like touching another person's feet? Do you therefore assume everyone else feels the same? Maybe you have ticklish feet and it is difficult for you when someone touches them, or maybe you fear encountering a fungus on a client's feet. You can see how the emotions associated with such beliefs can be problematic when giving a massage.

Issues like these can be overcome as therapists become more educated about problematic areas. For example, a therapist who is afraid of catching a fungus from a client can learn the signs and symptoms of potential problems and the universal precautions to take to prevent disease transmission. Learning to work on ticklish feet may be as simple as learning different approaches and pressures to apply.

It is not unusual for students to enter massage school without ever having received a professional massage. Most people have received some type of massage from a family member such as a mother or grandmother rubbing their shoulders or back when they were sore. We most likely have very good feelings and thoughts about this type of touch. It is generally agreed by most people that massage has many positive benefits for both the person receiving and the person giving a massage.

Most people believe that receiving massage feels very good and can alleviate painful areas. But "most" is not all, and many people have never had a professional massage and therefore may have mixed emotions or concerns. Those concerns may involve, for example, having a stranger rather than a friend or significant other give the massage. After answering the questions in Exercise 2-2, you may need to look within yourself to understand any issues you may have regarding bodywork. It is worthwhile to confront these issues now while still

a student. Working through your own concerns will help you better understand and work with your clients. Some of your clients may have the very same concerns that you have had.

Knowing what each type of massage and the techniques involved feels like will also help the person performing a massage relate to what a client is feeling. Can you imagine performing techniques without ever knowing what they feel like? Therapists could watch and think they know what it would feel like, but most professional therapists generally agree that what you see and feel can be different. Many details of massage are very subtle, and receiving a massage will help you "feel" what those little details are and why they may be important to a client. Clients will also report what they did or did not like about the draping or the environment of an office. Therapists may not realize how noisy an office is or that the draping was not tight enough until someone brings it to their attention. Many clients may not feel comfortable criticizing a therapist but instead will just find someone else to work on them.

Another benefit of receiving a professional massage is that it will help you understand what a client may feel like before the client's first massage. Clients often receive a gift certificate for a massage and may be concerned or have questions about the massage. Maybe the client is concerned about getting undressed or may have an issue with a certain part of his or her body. These are natural concerns for many people. As a professional, you want to make the session a very positive experience for all clients and have them return regularly. Working with your clients to address their concerns and meeting their needs is a very important part of being a massage professional.

Massages received from a professional as often as possible are a valuable learning tool. You can learn a great deal from other professionals while receiving a massage, and these massages will also help you take care of yourself. You will be recommending regular massages to your clients—doesn't it make sense to "practice what you preach"? It would be difficult to understand how particular techniques feel if you have not received the work yourself. Receiving massage from someone who has been practicing for many years can not only help you better realize the personal benefits of massage but can also give you valuable information about new skills, marketing ideas, and techniques that your clients might enjoy.

Most massage schools require that you both give and receive massages as part of the learning process. This is a wonderful part of your training in that you can experience the different types of techniques and skills with other students, and the feedback you

EXERCISE 2-2

If you have personal issues or fears that you do not want to discuss openly in class, write them down and talk to your instructor in private to work through them.

1. What are your concerns or reservations about receiving massage? _____

2. Do you have concerns about having someone else work on you? _____

3. How do you think you can address their concerns? _____

receive from others is valuable information for improving your work. Students need to experience all the touch therapies in order to process the information kinesthetically—for your body to understand it as well as your mind. Talk with your instructors if you are having difficulty with this aspect of training; they will understand and help you work through it. Most therapists at one time or another have been frustrated or did not like a particular type of massage. For example, you may at first not like giving a sports massage, but when you received the work yourself, you found that you benefited from the techniques.

Key Points

- It is common for students to have concerns about giving and receiving massage.
- Receiving massage from other professionals is a valuable learning tool.
- Receiving massage helps therapists relate to clients' concerns and questions.
- Address any concerns or questions with a mentor or your instructor.

THE CLIENT'S FEELINGS

Generally two types of individuals receive massage. The first have few if any reservations about receiving bodywork. Some may have received a great deal of work in the past and have no hesitation calling to make an appointment. Even with experienced clients, however, do not assume that their feelings will always be positive. For example, you have a new client who does not seem shy about receiving massage. You begin to work on her and everything goes well until you do some work on the upper leg and gluteal area. You suddenly notice that she is tensing up. You talk with the client, and she tells you she does not like to be touched in this area. Possibly you are the first massage therapist to work in this area. Communicating with clients about what you are doing is necessary, telling them what muscles are involved and why the work you are doing will help alleviate a symptom or problem. It is important to leave room for the client to communicate to you, and if the client continues to feel uncomfortable, leaving the area alone would show respect for the client's concerns. A client may also have some very strong emotional issues associated with a part of the body you are working on. Issues involving past abuse or neglect can suddenly arise while doing bodywork, often leaving the client feeling uncomfortable or vulnerable. A therapist should always be

conscious of a client's reaction to the work and work only within the client's comfort zone.

Other clients, typically with little or no massage experience, may be apprehensive about someone touching and working on them. Clients experience a wide array of feelings about what is appropriate in touch therapies. Some may feel uncomfortable disrobing for a massage, while others easily accept this. Some may—and should—feel that certain areas are out of bounds and should not be touched or worked on by a massage therapist. Some states have laws and regulations stipulating what areas are not to be touched, but clients' own feelings about areas of their bodies are equally if not more important than any state regulations. If you cross over the line of what the clients feels comfortable with, the client most likely will become emotional or tense. For example, you may feel that it is important to work the abdominal area, but some clients feel very vulnerable in this area and do not want to be touched there (Fig. 2-1). Their feelings may be related to an emotional protection or privacy issue. It is crucial to respect the client's needs for privacy. Even when you feel an area of the body needs work, it is the client who decides if and when the area will be worked. It is important to always address the client's needs and

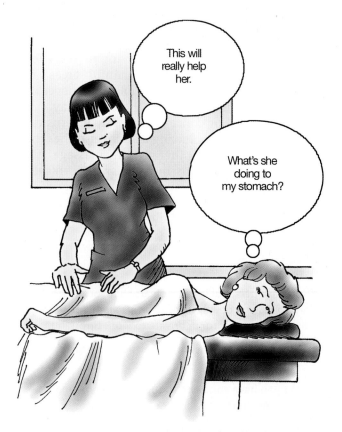

FIGURE 2-1 ■ **Your feelings about the massage may not be the same as the client's.** For example, not everyone feels comfortable with abdominal massage.

goals for a session. Pushing a technique or working on an area that a client does not like is not addressing the client's needs.

Signs that clients feel uncomfortable with a particular technique, pressure, or area being worked on include:

- Muscles tensing in other parts of the body
- Pulling the drape more tightly around them
- Fidgeting on the table
- Making a fist
- Holding their breath
- Talking nervously
- Bouncing their foot

All of these are signs that your client is in distress. Many clients do not feel comfortable telling you to stop but may simply lie there and endure the negative emotions they are feeling. As a professional bodyworker, you need to watch for these signs and communicate with the client to correct the situation. Even when asked, however, some clients may not feel comfortable telling you what is wrong. In this case, you can simply suggest stopping the work in that area or moving on to another area. If you do not pay attention to the signs of discomfort or you fail to check in with a client, the client may not return for another session. Such clients may not even be able to identify what they did not like about the session—but they will recall that they had some type of unpleasant feeling.

Clients' feelings about what they believe is right or wrong can be very strong. If a client believes that no work should be done on the abdomen, then that is the client's belief. If so, be very cautious about trying to convince the client to let you work on this area. If you think that working on the abdomen will help with a client's back pain, it is your responsibility to explain why you would do the work and how it has worked for other clients. Describing the technique and the benefits it offers gives clients the information necessary to make an educated choice about what they want or do not want in bodywork. Some clients may even take several sessions to decide they want to have a technique done. As clients gradually feel more comfortable with your work, they may trust you more to work in a vulnerable area.

The feelings of clients about being touched by another are one focus of the field of study now often called the psychology of touch. Many articles and books have addressed this issue. Elliott Greene and Barbara Greenwich-Dunn, in *The Psychology of the Body*, Elliott Greene, Barbara Greenwich-Dunn, Lippincott William and Wilkins; Baltimore, MD; 2004. explain that many psychological factors are involved in massage therapy. On the positive side, touch has several psychological roles:

- Touch is necessary for survival of infants and becomes associated with feelings of love, safety, and happiness.
- Touch is important for growth and development. But touch can also affect development negatively, such as when a child is punished by being slapped, spanked, or pinched; abusive touch can result in emotional scarring.
- Touch can promote emotional as well as physical healing.

Yet, as we have seen, touch can be perceived as threatening or intimidating by some clients, depending on their past experiences and feelings. It is crucial for massage therapists to understand the many possible dynamics involved in a client's feelings. For example, a client who has strong feelings about having the upper leg worked on may feel threatened; the client may become very emotional and may react by crying or becoming more tense, or may even ask you to stop the massage. Although you may think that area should be worked, the client may feel differently. The client may not feel like saying the area is sensitive to touch and could try instead to divert your attention to another part of the body. As a professional therapist, you must respect your clients' feelings about areas they do not want to be touched and their reasons why.

CASE STUDY

In her first appointment, Sara told the massage therapist that her back hurt but she had a hard time letting anyone work on it. She agreed to let the therapist try some light work on her upper back. As the therapist began to work, he noticed that her entire body tensed up whenever he touched her. The therapist asked if he was applying too much pressure, and at first Sara said it was okay. He told her he noticed that she was tensing up all over and asked if he should work on another area for a while. Sara said that it was really bothering her to have work done in this area right now and maybe he could just work on her legs for now.

After several sessions, Sara began to relax with the therapist and allowed him to work a little more each session on her back. Even though she was not completely relaxed, she was beginning to see the benefits of having her back worked on because it did decrease her physical pain. During her tenth session, she explained to the therapist that she had been mugged several years before and that her attacker had grabbed her from behind, hit her in the back, and held a knife to her throat. Sara said that she was seeing a psychologist and had discussed these issues with her. The psychologist explained to her how bodywork can cause the emotions associated with past physical events to resurface. Sara now felt comfortable enough to tell her massage therapist why she tensed up while he was working in certain areas.

Many clients may not feel comfortable telling their massage therapist information like this in their first sessions. But as they develop trust, they often begin to reveal information that helps the massage therapist make sense of their reactions. If a therapist feels a client is having difficulty coping with a response to bodywork, it is often good to refer the client to a psychologist, psychiatrist, or counselor.

Key Points

- Clients have different feelings about certain body areas.
- It is important to understand the apprehension clients may have.
- Respect the client's feelings and privacy.

Greene and Greenwich-Dunn also write about the many psychological elements affecting how clients respond to massage. Massage therapists, they write, should attempt to understand these aspects in their clients:

- A client's beliefs and values involve their roles and motivations, including if the client should take an active or passive role in the therapeutic relationship; should the therapist only help to facilitate the client's progress or take on a more authoritative role in the relationship?
- A client's expectations for the massage session may be consistent with or vary widely from the therapist's expectations.
- The client's personal history, of both massage therapy and touch in general, strongly affects his or her present attitudes and expectations.

All these factors are important as you work with the client, build trust, and establish a climate of emotional safety. These factors also help to build your professional reputation among clients, peers, and the community. Being proficient in massage techniques is a required part of the professional relationship, but equally important is how a therapist relates to a client in an emotional, nonphysical way.

WORKING WITH CLIENTS

ETHICS AND TRUST

Whenever you provide a service or product to the public, they expect it to be presented in an ethical way. When clients book an appointment for a massage, they naturally assume that your behavior will be ethical and they will feel safe while receiving a massage. Clients want to believe that you have high moral and ethical standards. Although they may not know much about you, they trust that they will be well taken care of as a client. Word of mouth is one of the most common ways that an individual becomes a client. People ask their friends, family, and co-workers about massage therapists they have seen, and they trust that these people will let them know who they can begin to trust as a therapist.

Trust is a very important issue in the massage community. You are asking clients to take off some or all of their clothing and have you touch parts of their body not usually touched by strangers (Fig. 2-2). If at any time the client begins to feel "unsafe," the client usually becomes very emotional or feels threatened. Clients who feel unsafe are not having their needs met and likely will not return for another session. You cannot assume that clients automatically know that you have only good intentions in mind for their massage—you have to earn their trust.

Clients expect you to act ethically according to their way of thinking, not yours. For example, how do you know precisely what a client's **"safety zone"** is? As discussed in Chapter 1, there are many differences in people's belief systems. Assuming that you always know what is good for a client can lead to problems in your practice.

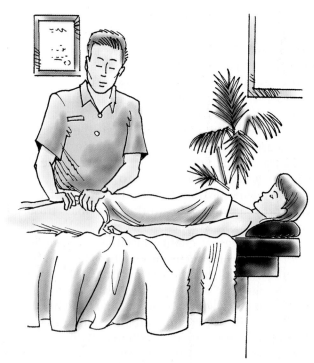

FIGURE 2-2 ■ A massage therapist must monitor the client's reaction to the massage.

EXERCISE 2-3

1. List six potential areas in which a person's beliefs and values could differ from yours.

_____

_____

2. Could any of these areas cause a potential problem in your practice? How?

_____

_____

3. What do you consider your own safety zone?

_____

4. How would you feel if someone else crossed what you consider your safety zone?

_____

5. How do you think you would react?

_____

Therapists should never assume they know what a client thinks or believes. The following sections will help you understand what a client has the right to believe and the importance of working with those beliefs. This is one way to earn a client's trust.

EMOTIONAL SAFETY

Remember that because of their past, your clients may have issues with certain aspects of being touched, and it is important to respect what feels right to them. For example, clients may have had siblings that frequently pestered them by tickling their feet. Clients may be sensitive to someone working on their feet because this made them uncomfortable.

Clients may choose not to tell you they have issues with parts of their bodies, or they may not even realize it until you touch the area. Either way, it is not ethical to pry into clients' feelings about their body. Because you are likely to encounter this type of situation, you should be prepared to handle it. First, it helps to be as informed as possible about the client's likes and dislikes through your **intake form** and the client interview. The more you know, the less likely it will be for a problem to arise unexpectedly in the middle of a session. Second, once a client has expressed a concern, either by saying something to you or by reacting in a way that you notice, it is your responsibility to be proactive in respecting the client's feelings and

wishes. If you ignore the situation and proceed with the massage, the client could feel that you have crossed over his or her personal boundaries. The client's needs should always be the focus of any session, even though a client may not always be aware of what those needs are at the beginning of a session. For example, if a client asks you to address a low back pain during a session, but while you are working on the area, the client begins to seem uneasy, it is best to check in with the client and assess whether work should continue in that area or you should move to another area.

It is not always easy to define what exactly makes a massage practice safe and ethical, and perceptions can vary between therapists and clients. Therapists who have been in practice for a number of years often are fairly comfortable with their values and beliefs and do not consciously have to think about what they do with every client. They instinctively know that they have to continually address the needs of the client and keep their focus on the session. A new therapist has to work at focusing on the client's needs along with the techniques during a session. Time and experience help a new therapist begin to feel more comfortable with not having to think about every variable of the session. The variables will begin to become part of who you are and what you do with each client. A therapist should be aware that a client is both receiving and giving information on a physical and mental level during a massage session.

It is also important to maintain a balance in the information you need. For example, in the earlier case study of Sara, it was good that the massage therapist learned that the client had an issue with her upper back, and knowing that she had been attacked helped the therapist make sense of her reaction. The therapist did not, however, need to know the details of the attack. He was not a psychotherapist treating the emotional aftermath of the attack but a bodyworker treating the physical effects of the attack in a positive and reinforcing way. It can be nurturing for clients to work with someone who is willing to help the healing process without being invasive.

COMMUNICATION

Before the first session begins with a new client, a professional massage therapist should know what the client's expectations are and any issues the client may have. You can learn this information in several ways.

Initial Contact

When a new client calls, that person begins checking you out almost immediately. The prospective client may ask for information about the services you offer, such as price, the different types of massage you perform, and other general questions. The person will listen to your tone of voice and want to be reassured that you are a good and safe therapist to make an appointment with. If you seem unsure of yourself or give vague answers, the caller may not feel comfortable making an appointment. If you have a receptionist or others in your workplace who answer the phones and make appointments, make sure they are fully trained to answer questions as well as know how to build trust with clients. Some businesses fail to train receptionists or telephone staff adequately, and their information can easily be wrong or give clients the wrong impression. You can imagine how misinformation could be problematic in a massage practice.

For example, in a massage therapy school students were asked to research the services being provided in the area where they would be opening their practices. Students reported back to the class what they were told, and talked about how some receptionists and therapists did not do a good job answering their questions. One student had asked what type of Oriental sessions were offered. The receptionist told her they had "Shitzu therapy." (Obviously she should have said Shiatsu—not Shitzu like the breed of dog!) These students quickly learned the value of therapists educating the person who talks to the public on their behalf.

Client Intake Form

On your intake form, it is good to ask clients what their goals are for their massage session(s) (Fig 2-3). You may have assumed a client wants a relaxation massage, for example, when actually he or she wants pain relief from a recent back injury. Just as important are questions about areas where clients do not want work. You can include on your intake form a list of areas for clients to check off those they do or do not want worked on. This allows your clients to easily indicate what they feel comfortable with and helps prevent situations in which you might make incorrect assumptions or have to ask about things the client may be uncomfortable talking about. Alternatively, a diagram of the body can be used to allow clients to mark areas they do or do not want included in the massage.

It is also very important to note, that some states require that certain information be obtained from each client. Be sure to check on your state's laws and regulations regarding information that may be required, and include this as part of your health history or client intake form.

Client Interview

The client interview is an important step in building trust with a client. Many clients are surprised about the amount of information that massage therapists request on a health intake form. Begin by explaining the form to the client, including reading any disclosures the client should sign. There are two schools of thought about how to conduct an interview. The first is to leave the client alone while filling out the form. This gives the client some time to think about the information requested. Other therapists feel more comfortable being with the client when the form is filled out and asking questions about the client's health. There is no one right way to do the client interview, as long as therapists choose what they feel is the best way to gather the needed information.

If your client is filling out the form, it is important to sit down and discuss and clarify any concerns related to the health history. For example, the client may have put down a medication that is not familiar to you. Asking the client what the medication is for can give you additional information about the client's health. An important question to ask either on the health history form or verbally is the client's goal for the session. Most clients have at least a general idea of what they want to achieve during a massage. Knowing the client's stated intention helps a therapist know what direction the massage should take. If several different types of treatment could meet that goal, it is good to discuss these options at this time with the client. At the end of interview, before the session begins, restate the goals for the session.

The time it takes to interview a client may depend on the client's current health. If a client has recently had a health concern or has a number of health conditions that should be discussed, the interview could take up to 15 to 20 minutes. Some clients are anxious to tell you everything about their health, while others are somewhat wary of giving you personal information. Explaining why you need to know certain information for their own safety helps reassure clients that you are not just being nosy. Taking the time to evaluate what type of work should be done due to a client's health is an important responsibility for all therapists. If a client is fairly healthy and lists only a few things on the health history, the interview process can take only a few minutes.

Careful Observation and Focus on the Client

Therapists should pay close attention to clients from the time they walk in the door until they leave. When you greet them on their arrival, you'll already

Client Intake Form

Name _____ Date _____

Address _____

City, State, Zip _____

Phone (Day) _____ (Evening) _____

Where did you hear about us? _____

Reason for your visit _____

Health History

Medications you are currently taking: (Please include over-the-counter medications)

_____

Reason for taking above medication(s): _____

Please list any surgeries and the approximate date:

_____

Please indicate if you have had any of the following conditions:

___Headaches   ___Seizures   ___Sinus infection   ___Concussions

___Fractures   ___Back pain   ___Neck pain   ___Arthritis

___Asthma   ___Swelling   ___Fainting   ___Heart disease

___Skin rash   ___Numbness   ___Joint disease   ___Digestive disease

___Blood clots   ___Allergies   ___Cancer   ___High or low blood pressure

Please list any medical conditions you may have that are not listed above. *It is important that your therapist be informed about all medical conditions, because massage can make some conditions worse. All information is confidential.*

_____

_____

During your massage session, the therapist may be working on the following parts of your body, always using appropriate draping for your safety and comfort. Please check any areas you do **not** feel comfortable having the therapist work on.

__Neck ___Shoulder __Back __Arms __Legs __ Chest __ Abdomen __Feet __ Gluteals

I have informed the therapist of all conditions I am currently aware of and attest that this information is accurate and true. Therapists will not prescribe any medications, will not perform any spinal manipulations, and will work within their scope of practice, abiding by all laws, rules, and regulations that apply. Please sign and date below.

_____   _____

Client Signature   **Date**

FIGURE 2-3 ■ Example of a client intake form.

be getting a general sense of what state the client is in. If they have having a rough day or they are apprehensive about receiving a massage, you will be able to see those emotions if you pay close attention. Educating a new client about the massage session and the room will also help an apprehensive client relax and feel more comfortable. Educate the client about how they will be draped for the session. Explain that you will ask them occasionally about how comfortable they are, but they should feel free to speak up at any time if the pressure is too heavy or too light, if they feel chilled, or if they have any other concerns. Explain the general pattern of the massage routine you will be using. This will keep clients from wondering what the therapist will be doing next. Let clients know how to position themselves on the table and what coverings you will be using. Also reassure clients that they will have plenty of time to get ready for the massage and you will knock before entering the room. During the massage, keep observing the client for any sign of distress, such as tensing up, bouncing a foot, or fidgeting on the table.

After the Session

After completing the session, tell the client you are leaving the room. Instruct clients to get up slowly, in case they feel a little dizzy or light-headed. Explain to the client how to get off the table. Explain to clients where to go after they have dressed. Leave the room, but stay close enough to hear in case a client calls for assistance. Check in with clients to see how they feel and if they have any questions. This is also a good time to explain to a client the after effects of the massage. For example, if work was done on a problem area, the client could have some soreness the next day. This is also the time to give any additional information or homework to a client. During the session, if you have suggested that the client stretch a particular area, this is the time to either show the client how to do that or to provide information on the stretches.

Some facilities have a client fill out an evaluation form. It is best to keep this short and to the point. Asking simple yes-or-no questions is best to allow the client to give feedback. A place for comments at the bottom of the form lets clients who want to say more express their thoughts. If appropriate, book another appointment with the client and be sure to write down in your notes any client concerns or questions for their next session.

All of these suggestions and ideas should help you assure your clients that their safety and well-being are important in your practice. Any therapist who does not use a health history form or ask clients about their needs and preferences is not

---

EXERCISE 2-4

1. Write a script explaining your massage routine to a client. _____

2. Practice your script so that you can follow it without using your notes. _____

3. Present your script to the class. (Use props as needed, such as a massage table.)

---

doing a professional job. It is critical to know what a client's health is, because many health conditions contraindicate a massage. Clients will return to a therapist with whom they feel safe but will rarely book another session with a therapist who performs massage simply to earn a paycheck.

CHARACTERISTICS OF SUCCESS

Successful bodyworkers will tell you that treating clients ethically is one of the most important features of their practice. Following are some additional important components for having a successful relationship with your clients.

1. Professionally communicate with your clients. You should know enough about their health to safely treat them. But if too much discussion is taking place about a condition, the relationship may become more personal than professional. Some clients may want to give you the entire story, for example, about the car accident that affected their back.

2. It is your responsibility to ask for information that will help you treat clients effectively. You should know what would make the client feel uncomfortable. For example, the client may have ticklish feet.

3. If a conflict does arise, address it immediately. If a client is visibly upset, ask about it right away and try to resolve the problem. Respect the clients' rights and feelings and do not pry into their personal issues.

4. Be proactive. Gather the information you need to treat your client safely and effectively. Inform the client about the treatments and modalities you will be using.

5. When in doubt about a client's needs, ask a mentor in your field for help. Respect your client's privacy by not disclosing identifiable personal information. Discuss the situation with your mentor to find the appropriate action to take.

6. Always keep the client's safety and trust in the forefront of your thoughts.

Key Points

- A client's trust in a massage therapist is crucial.
- Your massage practice should feel emotionally safe for your clients.
- Effective communication clarifies the client's expectations.
- Clients will trust a therapist who works toward their goals in massage sessions.

SUMMARY

It is perfectly normal for people to be emotional about their personal beliefs, values, and ethics. As a massage therapist, you should have strong feelings about being ethical in your practice. As you become still more aware and knowledgeable about professional ethics and behavior, you will see even more value and importance in understanding what your clients believe and feel. Take ownership of your ethics, and these principles will become a strong foundation for your practice. Clients will feel your strong foundation and good ethical makeup. They will feel safe and trust your professionalism. You will enjoy the benefits of emotional safety in your work while you build a great practice.

Never forget that clients will come to you with a wide variety of beliefs and values that may be quite different from your own. Be nonjudgmental and flexible as you work with these beliefs. If a client expresses or acts on a belief or value not in keeping with your professional ethics, as we will see in later chapters, you have the right not to accept or keep this person as a client. The safety of both your clients and you as the practitioner should always be foremost and is the basis for the professional ethical codes you will learn about in the next chapter.

ADDITIONAL ACTIVITIES

With the class divided into two groups, one group should write questions or requests that clients potentially have before or during a massage session. Present these to the other group, who should then answer or demonstrate what the group members should do in each situation. Then the class should discuss other ways these questions could be answered or addressed.

3

CODE OF ETHICS

CHAPTER PREVIEW

- Importance of professional ethics for therapists and clients
- Codes of ethics for the massage therapy profession
- Applying codes of ethics in a massage therapy practice
- Regulating ethical behavior

KEY TERMS

Code of ethics: a document stating an individual's or group's beliefs, standards, and ethical expectations

Professional ethics: a consensus of a group or association about its expectations concerning ethical principles and behavior

Scope of practice: a definition or set of parameters for activities a professional is or is not allowed to perform as defined by one's competency, training, and laws and regulations

Self-regulation: process by which a group, association, or profession sets guidelines, expectations, and repercussions for inappropriate behavior

Standards of practice: accepted way in which ethical behavior is performed

Most businesses, groups, and organizations understand the importance of having a document that states their values and beliefs about ethical behavior and expectations. This document is called a **code of ethics.** An association's code of ethics puts its beliefs and values into public view for members of the association and anyone who may be considering using a professional from that group. The code of ethics helps individuals and group members conduct their business in a way that the profession considers ethical. The code may also help form the guidelines for how a professional may act when faced with a situation in which an ethical decision is needed. A code of ethics has guidelines for many situations and is often particularly useful for an individual who is new in the profession and who has not faced situations that may require an ethical decision. No one can know in advance what to do in every possible situation, but having these basic guidelines to follow can be very helpful.

Your professional ethics, as discussed in the preceding chapters, may be very similar to your **professional ethics,** but there may also be some marked differences, as you will discover in this chapter.

FROM PERSONAL TO PROFESSIONAL ETHICS

As you examined your own personal beliefs, values, and morals in the previous chapters, you realized the importance of being aware of your own ethics for your practice of massage and bodywork. You take ownership of your personal code of right and wrong. Your personal knowledge and awareness will assist you when a situation arises in which you need to make an ethical decision. Taking steps to bring this awareness to the forefront is an important part of becoming a successful practitioner in the bodywork profession. Some members of the general public may still have some reservations about bodywork because of the past associations with illegal practices and the fact that massage is a very personal undertaking for those that receive it. How the public perceives your ethics or lack of ethics can be important for your success in the massage profession.

If all practitioners wrote their own personal codes of ethics, there would be some similarities, but there might also be some differences or gray areas. The very nature of personal ethics means some areas are subjective. Draping practices are an example of such differences. The general principle of providing draping that ensures the client's safety and privacy may be interpreted differently by two different therapists. How you choose to drape may be influenced by your own feelings of what feels safe and provides privacy, and that could be different from what someone else feels is safe and private. A professional code, however, helps resolve such differences.

Another example involves the right to refuse a client for just and reasonable cause. If a client makes a slightly off-color remark, is that enough of a reason to refuse to treat him or her? Some therapists may feel threatened by such remarks, while other may feel they can handle the situation. If a client were to react negatively to being refused treatment, the massage therapist can refer to a code of ethics and explain that inappropriate remarks are a just cause for refusing treatment.

After professional associations and groups initially formed in the bodywork community, it was not long before these associations realized that they needed to present the public and potential members with a statement of their belief and value system. Documents expressing a code of ethics were written to show potential members the expectations of the group for ethical conduct. These codes also demonstrated to the public what ethical standards group members are expected to maintain for behavior. Groups and associations in the massage community have long felt the need for safe and effective training for their members and for telling the public what they should expect from a professional bodyworker. Therefore, they formulated guidelines for their members to follow. These guidelines also define inappropriate behavior. If a client makes a complaint against one of the group's members, these guidelines help the association determine if the massage therapist in fact did something wrong. Although all individuals have their own beliefs about what is right or wrong, the professional association's code of ethics reflects a consensus of what the group feels is right and wrong. Two such codes

of ethics are shown here, from the American Massage Therapy Association (AMTA) and the National Certification Board for Therapeutic Massage and Bodywork (NCBTMB). Codes from other groups and associations are presented later in the chapter.

American Massage Therapy Association Code of Ethics

This Code of Ethics is a summary statement of the standards by which massage therapists agree to conduct their practices and is a declaration of the general principles of acceptable, ethical and professional behavior.

Massage therapists shall:

1. Demonstrate a commitment to provide the highest quality massage therapy/bodywork to those who seek their professional service.
2. Acknowledge the inherent worth and individuality of each person by not discriminating or behaving in any prejudicial manner with clients and/or colleagues.
3. Demonstrate professional excellence through regular self-assessment of strengths, limitations and effectiveness by continued education and training.
4. Acknowledge the confidential nature of the professional relationship with clients and respect each client's right to privacy.
5. Conduct all business and professional activities within their scope of practice, the law of the land, and project a professional image.
6. Refrain from engaging in any sexual conduct or sexual activities involving their clients.
7. Accept responsibility to do no harm to the physical, mental and emotional well-being of self, clients and associates.

The National Certification Board for Therapeutic Massage and Bodywork Code of Ethics

The Code of Ethics of the National Certification Board for Therapeutic Massage and Bodywork (NCBTMB) requires certificants to uphold professional standards that allow for the proper discharge of their responsibilities to those served, that protect the integrity of the profession, and that safeguard the interest of individual clients. Those practitioners who have been awarded national certification by the NCBTMB will:

- Have the sincere commitment to provide the highest quality of care to those that seek their professional services.
- Represent their qualifications honestly, including their educational achievements and profes-

sional affiliations, and will provide only those services which they are qualified to perform.

- Accurately inform clients, other health care practitioners, and the public of the scope and limitations of their discipline. Acknowledge the limitations of and contraindications for massage and bodywork and refer clients to appropriate health professionals.
- Provide treatment only where there is reasonable expectation that it will be advantageous to the client.
- Consistently maintain professional knowledge and competence, striving for professional excellence through regular assessment of personal and professional strengths and weaknesses and through continued education training.
- Conduct their business and professional activities with honesty and integrity, and respect the inherent worth of all persons.
- Refuse to unjustly discriminate against clients and other health professionals.
- Safeguard the confidentiality of all client information, unless disclosure is required by law, court order, or is absolutely necessary for the protection of the public.
- Respect the client's right to treatment and informed and voluntary consent. The NCBMTB practitioner will obtain and record the informed consent of the client, or client's advocate, before providing treatment. This consent may be written or verbal.
- Respect the client's right to refuse, modify or terminate treatment regardless of prior consent given.
- Provide draping and treatment in a way that ensures the safety, comfort and privacy of the client.
- Exercise the right to refuse to treat any person or part of the body for just and reasonable cause.
- Refrain, under all circumstances, from initiating or engaging in any sexual conduct, sexual activities, or sexualizing behavior involving a client, even if the client attempts to sexualize the relationship.
- Avoid any interest, activity or influence which might be in conflict with the practitioner's obligation to act in the best interest of the client or the profession.
- Respect the client's boundaries with regard to privacy, disclosure, exposure, emotional expression, beliefs, and the client's reasonable expectations of professional behavior. Practitioners will respect the client's autonomy.
- Refuse any gifts or benefits which are intended to influence a referral, decision or treatment that are purely for personal gain and not for the good of the client.
- Follow all policies, procedures, guidelines, regulations, codes, and requirements promulgated by the National Certification Board of Therapeutic Massage and Bodywork.

WHY PROFESSIONAL ETHICS ARE IMPORTANT

Professional ethics are the standards that members of that professional agree to adhere to. Most professions have general rules that most members of the profession agree are important and should be followed. The application of general guidelines in every situation, however, often involves some interpretation of these guidelines. That is why most associations in the bodywork profession have developed a code of ethics to which members of these associations are expected to adhere.

A code of ethics is a living document in the sense that it is always being scrutinized for any changes that may be needed. As the guidelines are tested in the practice of bodywork, an association may see the need to change its code to help members better understand the expectations. An example of this is the wording in codes involving therapists disclosing information regarding their training and the effects of the different types of modalities that they offer. More than 100 massage modalities are now available to the public, and the associations ask that their members truthfully explain what type of training they have had and the expected effects of the client's session(s). You may have heard that, in general, rules are written because someone has done something wrong. This is also true of associations and the codes they write and adopt. Some of those guidelines have been written because some people have crossed a line into what most in the profession consider to be unacceptable behavior.

On the positive side, guidelines can offer assistance or structure that may be needed if an ethical decision is required. For example, if your client asks you to perform a chiropractic adjustment on his neck while doing a massage, a simple answer is that it is ethically, or in some cases legally, beyond your **scope of practice** to perform that type of technique. Clients can readily understand such an answer. Such questions arise because the general public often does not understand where the scope of practice for a bodyworker begins and ends, especially with all the different types of alternative therapies available today.

THE IMPORTANCE OF PROFESSIONAL CODES FOR BODYWORKERS

The guidelines and structure of a professional code of ethics helps bodyworkers know what behaviors are expected and are useful when you must make decisions in your practice. You can refer to the code of ethics if a client questions why you have made a certain decision or behave in a particular way. For example, if your client says she does not care if you stay in the room while she disrobes, you might first say that you feel better leaving the room to give her privacy. If the client still does not understand this concept, you can point out that it is against your professional code of ethics—which makes a very clear statement to the client.

The code of ethics is therefore a safety net for bodyworkers when situations arise in which you cannot quickly or easily think of how to explain your behavior or decision to a client. In the example above, changing the uncomfortable situation into a simple ethical issue states the case in a way that a client would have a hard time arguing against. As a new practitioner, you may find it difficult sometimes to give a quick, confident answer to a client's question or request. With a professional code of ethics, however, you can confidently give the client a valid, specific answer as to why you may or may not do something. Most, if not all, bodyworkers have faced ethical questions in their practice, and with time you too will feel confident with your answers to a client's requests. Your own comfort level will increase with time and experience, but in the beginning of your practice, you can rely on your association's code of ethics to give you the initial structure that you need.

CASE STUDY

A female bodyworker has had regular sessions with a male client for about 6 months when he begins to ask her personal questions. He asks if she has a boyfriend and says he'd like to take her out sometime. She tries to avoid his questions as best she can and tries to change the subject and continue with the session. Over the next few sessions, however, he continues to ask more about her personal life. It is getting hard for her to avoid this conversation. He finally asks if she would like to have dinner with him soon. She tells the client that it is against her profession's code of ethics to become personally involved with a client and that she will not go out with him as long as he is a client. This answer lets the client know that the professional code encompasses what she as a therapist can and cannot do.

The general public has high expectations about receiving services from professionals, but often the public does not consider that professionals also have expectations for how they are treated by the public. Often clients do not stop to think that they may have requested something that is inappropriate. The earlier example of a client asking for a chiropractic adjustment can be an innocent request from a client who does not know that bodyworkers are not trained to do this type of procedure.

EXERCISE 3-1

Look over the four codes presented in this chapter.

1. Pick out three individual codes that you feel would be easy for you to follow and adhere to. List your reasons.

_____

_____

2. Are there any items in any of the codes that you feel uneasy with or do not understand how you will comply? List your reasons.

_____

_____

3. Have a class discussion regarding the codes that seem clearly defined and would be easy to follow. Discuss with the class which code statements may present some challenges. As a group, come up with alternative wording or solutions of how to follow the codes.

_____

_____

Key Points
- Professional ethics provide structure and guidelines.
- Professional ethics provide safety for practitioners.
- Professional ethics are written into codes that can be shown to clients when needed.

THE IMPORTANCE OF PROFESSIONAL CODES FOR CLIENTS

A segment of the U.S. population continues to scrutinize the practice of bodywork and massage. People in many other countries generally do not have a problem with accepting massage as a legitimate profession. In the United States, however, the sex trade for a long time used the word "massage" to refer to illegal practices such as prostitution and other sexual services, and some in the general public still raise an eyebrow when people say they perform massage therapy for a living. The media have done a very good job of showing the positive sides and the true meaning of the massage profession over the last 10 years, but it is still important that we continue to demonstrate to the public that bodywork professionals follow professional ethics.

The public, who are your clients, need to trust that they will be treated in a professional manner. This means that they need to trust that we will perform only the bodywork techniques we are trained to do. How would you feel if a doctor performed a type of surgery on you in which he or she had little or no training? The same holds true for all the different types of bodywork. The public wants to know that you are a skilled practitioner in the types of therapies that you offer.

The public also needs to know that they will be treated with respect. This means that you will listen to the client's needs or goals for the session and not simply do what you want or feel like doing. For example, if your client tells you that he has pain in his upper back and neck and would just like to have a relaxing massage, it would be inappropriate to perform deep tissue or trigger point therapy during the session without his permission. It is not appropriate to perform a modality on your client without discussing it with him first. There have been many cases in which clients have requested a certain type of work or goal for the massage and the therapist ignored the request or did not do as requested and clients left the session feeling like their issues or needs were not addressed. Clients request a service or goal and will trust a therapist who meets their needs.

Clients usually do not ask for your code of ethics when making an appointment. They may see it in your brochure or posted in your office. Often clients are referred to you by a person or client who feels you are a good therapist. Part of being a good therapist is having a strong ethical makeup.

Key Points

- Clients want to trust their therapist.
- Ethical structure and guidelines help clients know expectations for both the client and the therapist.
- Ethics become part of who you are as a professional.

PROFESSIONALISM AND ETHICS

Professionalism and ethics seem to go hand in hand in the business world today. You cannot turn on the television or read a newspaper without hearing about something that a business or person has done that is illegal or unethical. Criminal charges and lawsuits are being filed in record numbers these days because of such behaviors. Criminal charges are usually filed when an individual or business has done something that is against the law. Lawsuits can be filed in cases when laws have been broken and someone is looking for compensation or the law does not cover an issue and a possible ethical issue has arisen. Unfortunately, there have been cases where criminal charges have been filed against someone doing massage, mainly when sexual activities were involved. Lawsuits have been filed for damages when a client felt that he or she had been injured or damaged in some way during a massage session. It is important for bodyworkers to know what laws, rules, and regulations pertain to their profession.

Ethics are the highest standards that a person or a profession can follow. Laws state what is wrong or right to do, but an unethical person may "bend" or work around the law or use loopholes or technicalities to work things to their advantage. A professional who is serious about having a good reputation, however, will not look for loopholes to get around the law but will work within professional guidelines to provide ethical services.

DEVELOPING A CODE OF ETHICS

Most professions have developed a code of ethics that can be referred to by all parties as the guidelines and expectations for its members or professionals (Fig. 3-1). For example, when an association has a code of ethics and someone questions the behavior of a member of that association, the code of ethics is used to determine if that member did or did not do something unethical. Without a code of ethics, it would be a more difficult and subjective task for the group to decide right and wrong behavior. Most groups or associations used a process of **self-regulation** to evaluate, on the basis of their code of ethics, any complaints that are received. Associations and professions use their codes of ethics continuously in this important way.

In addition to a code of ethics, some groups and associations develop other documents such as **standards of practice.** These standards are an expanded, more specific version of the code of ethics that can help identify and define all elements in the code and fill in areas that might otherwise be open to subjective interpretation. Standards offer more specific definition

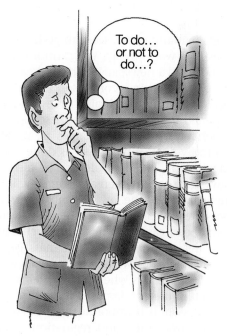

FIGURE 3-1 ■ Consult your professional association's code of ethics whenever you are in doubt about something.

and explanation of the expectations contained in a code. For example, a code may state that clients are to be treated in a sanitary facility, and the standards will describe specifically how a facility is to be maintained in this way. Use of a 10% bleach solution for cleaning and sanitizing, storage specifications for materials, and following universal precautions (precautions recommended for all health care providers) are all examples of specific guidelines in standards of practice. If any aspect of the code of ethics can be interpreted in several different ways, the standards of practice will generally provide a more concrete structure to follow.

Standards of practice may or may not be part of an association's documentation. If you are a member of an association and need further explanation about anything in the code of ethics or standards, you can contact the group for clarification.

A profession's scope of practice, however, is different from the standards of practice. Scope of practice is a legal definition or set of parameters for activities a professional is or is not allowed to perform. State laws, rules, or regulations may define the scope of practice for massage therapists. A professional organization can also define what it deems is appropriate for a member to practice. The legal definitions usually very specifically describe the techniques and skills a therapist can perform. If a therapist were to practice outside that scope, the legal repercussions set down by the state could result. For example, if the scope of practice states that no spinal manipulations will be performed and a therapist deliberately adjusted someone's back, the client would have the legal right

to file a complaint with the state agency or board. All therapists should know their scope of practice and know the implications for practicing outside that scope of practice.

> **Key Points**
> ■ Most professions develop a code of ethics to define expectations for the public and its members.
> ■ A code of ethics changes as the profession or members of a group deem necessary.
> ■ Standards of practice help to define the specific guidelines of a code of ethics.
> ■ A scope of practice defines what a therapist can and cannot do.

HOW ASSOCIATIONS WRITE A CODE OF ETHICS

As associations or groups form, the individuals who help organize them soon realize the need for ground rules or guidelines to help the group and its members practice efficiently. Some groups begin with very simple documents, while others may start out with a lengthy code. Often a small core group of people works on a document to present to a board of directors or to the members for approval. A code of ethics is usually considered a living document, which means that changes are made when a group deems there is a need.

The American Massage Therapy Association (AMTA) is a member-driven organization of massage therapists. The National Board of Directors oversees a number of committees that work on documents such as the code of ethics or standards of practice when the board determines that work is needed on these documents. Many groups review their documents every few years or on an as-need basis. If something within the code seems not to be working or is being interpreted in different ways, the group may go back to work to define the expectations more clearly.

A code of ethics is a very public document for many groups. It is a statement of what they believe and their expectations for their members. Every member is given a copy of the code of ethics, and after joining the group each member is expected to follow the code's guidelines. The code of ethics is available to the general public through advertising and marketing materials, requests for information, and Internet sites. It is easy to understand why so many groups spend a great deal of time on this document to ensure the public has the correct perception of their profession.

Associated Bodywork and Massage Professionals (ABMP) Professional Code of Ethics

As a member of Associated Bodywork and Massage Professionals, I hereby pledge to abide by the ABMP Code of Ethics as outlined below.

Client Relationships

■ I shall endeavor to serve the best interest of my clients at all times and to provide the highest quality service possible.

■ I shall maintain clear and honest communications with my clients and shall keep client communications confidential.

■ I shall acknowledge the limitations of my skills and, when necessary, refer clients to the appropriate qualified health care professional.

■ I shall in no way instigate or tolerate any kind of sexual advance while acting in the capacity of a massage, bodywork, somatic therapy or esthetic practitioner.

Professionalism

■ I shall maintain the highest standards of professional conduct, providing services in an ethical and professional manner in relation to my clientele, business associates, health care professionals, and the general public.

■ I shall respect the rights of all ethical practitioners and will cooperate with all health care professionals in a friendly and professional manner.

■ I shall refrain from the use of any mind-altering drugs, alcohol, or intoxicants prior to or during professional sessions.

■ I shall always dress in a professional manner, proper dress being defined as attire suitable and consistent with accepted business and professional practice.

■ I shall not be affiliated with or employed by any business that utilizes any form of sexual suggestiveness or explicit sexuality in its advertising or promotion of services, or in the actual practice of its services.

Scope of Practice/Appropriate Techniques

■ I shall provide services within the scope of the ABMP definition of massage, bodywork, somatic therapies and skin care, and the limits of my training. I will not employ those massage, bodywork, or skin care techniques for which I have not had adequate training and shall represent my education, training, qualifications and abilities honestly.

■ I shall be conscious of the intent of the services that I am providing and shall be aware of and practice good judgment regarding the application of massage, bodywork or somatic techniques utilized.

■ I shall not perform manipulations or adjustments of the human skeletal structure, diagnose, prescribe or provide any other service, procedure or therapy which requires a license to practice chiropractic, osteopathy, physical therapy, podiatry, orthopedics, psychotherapy, acupuncture, dermatology, cosmetology, or any other profession or branch of medicine unless specifically licensed to do so.

■ I shall be thoroughly educated and understand the physiological effects of specific massage, bodywork, somatic or skin care techniques utilized in order to determine whether such application is contraindicated and/or to determine the most beneficial techniques to apply to a given individual. I shall not apply massage, bodywork, somatic or skin care techniques in those cases where they may be contraindicated without a written referral from the client's primary care provider.

Image/Advertising Claims

■ I shall strive to project a professional image for myself, my business or place of employment, and the profession in general.

■ I shall actively participate in educating the public regarding the actual benefits of massage, bodywork, somatic therapies and skin care.

■ I shall practice honestly in advertising, promote my services ethically and in good taste, and practice and/or advertise only those techniques for which I have received training and/or certification. I shall not make false claims regarding the potential benefits of the techniques rendered.

Ontario Massage Therapy Association Code of Ethics

Preamble

The ethical foundation of the practice of Massage Therapy consists of moral obligations which ensure the dignity and integrity of the profession.

The aim of the Code is to define clearly those obligations and those professional duties which must be observed by every practitioner and also to define some of the major and minor abuses which must be avoided.

Study of the Code should develop in every student and every practitioner a highly sensitive professional conscience. It is the imperative duty of every Massage Therapist to adhere strictly not only to the regulations prescribed by the Code of Ethics, but equally to its moral precepts.

In addition to the items covered in the Code of Ethics, every Massage Therapist should be cognizant of and must abide by the regulations of the Regulated Health Professions Act and the Massage Therapy Act as they pertain to Massage Therapy.

Section 1 Service to the Public

1. The Massage Therapist's first duty is to the public.
2. The Therapist should inform the patient of fees, and the type of treatment recommended prior to such treatment.
3. When it is necessary in the interest of the patient, the Therapist should recommend that the patient seek expert medical advice.
4. A Therapist must respect the confidence of the patient, not discussing the patient by name without his or her consent.
5. A Therapist's establishment must be clean and neat.
6. Linens and towels must be laundered before each use with another patient.
7. On the patient's request, the Therapist must render a receipt for all monies paid.
8. A Therapist must not make unreasonable or unsubstantiated claims regarding massage generally or his or her techniques specifically.

Section 2 Service to the Public

A Therapist must not make disparaging remarks concerning the practices, abilities or competence of other Massage Therapists or about practitioners in other health disciplines.

Notwithstanding the above, where a member of this Association is aware and has proof of the misconduct of, breach of trust or other violation or transgression of this Code of Ethics by any member of this Association, it is his or her duty to bring such knowledge and proof to the attention of the Board of Directors of this Association.

Section 3 Records

The Therapist must maintain accurate and up-to-date records of the dates and types of treatment given to each patient, and fees charged.

SIMILARITIES AND DIFFERENCES IN CODES

The codes of ethics included in this chapter are from several different associations and groups in the massage and bodywork field. As you read through the different codes, you will notice that most codes address certain key areas such as the scope of practice, referrals, appearance, confidentiality, respect, and knowledge. Some code statements are very specific, while others may leave room for some interpretation. Some similarities include requirements that therapists:

- Maintain confidentiality of clients
- Be committed to high quality care and the best interest of clients
- Continue education
- Respect clients
- Refer clients when needed
- Make accurate claims about types of modalities
- Not sexualize massage and bodywork

As you read through the codes, you will notice the focus of each one. In some, respect for the client's needs, confidentiality, and integrity are foremost. In others, specific expectations for therapist are more obvious. Each group or association that formulated these codes had its own reasons to put its codes in writing. The authors of these codes also had strong feelings about what is needed in the bodywork profession. Some may have felt that clients had been taken advantage of and that strong guidelines were needed to protect clients. Others may have felt that bodyworkers needed more stringent guidelines in order to be successful. All of the codes contain important and pertinent information for use by therapists and clients, and almost all of the codes cover certain key issues. Several of the codes draw clear-cut lines regarding sexual contact and involvement between clients and the therapist. These statements help prevent any subjective interpretation of such conduct.

EXERCISE 3-2

1. Read through the four codes of ethics again. Make a check mark beside every statement that is clearly defined and leaves little or no room for interpretation.
2. Place an X by any statement that is not clearly defined and leaves room for interpretation or questions.
3. How could you restate any code statements you marked with an X to make them more clearly understood?
4. Do you feel all code statements should be included in your own personal code? If not, which would you not include? Why?

_____

_____

_____

_____

REGULATION OF ETHICAL PRACTICES

THERAPIST MISBEHAVIOR

A code of ethics can be a working document for a group or association to assist members and the general public to know the guidelines and expectations for bodyworkers. When a member of a group does something that a client feels is inappropriate, the client has the right to file a complaint against the therapist. Clients may or may not already have a copy of the code that the therapist should follow, but they may then seek out the code and may find that there has been a violation. The client can contact the therapist's association and learn the process by which a complaint is made. Sometimes a client may instead contact the local police, city hall, state board or agency, or even a business association if he does not know what else to do. Clients may also tell other therapists what happened and ask them for assistance or guidance. In other cases, they may simply drop the issue and be left with a bad opinion about the profession of massage and bodywork.

Most groups, associations, and state agencies have policies and procedures for filing a complaint. Most have a grievance committee for complaints that will follow a set procedure to handle a complaint. Rarely is a complaint handled by only one person within a group. Confidentiality is an important component of this process, along with obtaining legal advice about how to handle the complaint. A client may even feel the need to file a lawsuit against a therapist.

A group or agency may take a variety of actions on a complaint. These actions are generally clearly stated in the group's policies, procedures, or bylaws. Actions may include a warning letter, suspension, revocation of a membership or license, or dropping the complaint. Both parties will be informed of any action that is taken.

The American Massage Therapy Association has the Commission on Grievances that handles complaints made against its members. The commission has a set procedure for submitting and reviewing complaints. Appropriate legal issues and the code of ethics are considered when reviewing the complaint. It is important for all bodyworkers to know about the processes for such actions when joining a group or association and when working under state laws and regulations.

CLIENT MISBEHAVIOR

Clients are not regulated by the groups or associations of bodyworkers. When a client misbehaves, the therapist has cause to be concerned and can turn to his or her professional or personal code of ethics for guidance in handling the situation. Any client who tries to make a therapist act unethically should not be kept as a client. If a client innocently asks you to do something that is against your code of ethics, simply state what your policy or code is, and most clients will realize that they have crossed a boundary. If the client continues to request something that is unethical, you may need to let the client go. Depending on the situation, a therapist may need to end a session and not schedule any further appointments. Many codes and regulations state that a therapist may choose not to treat a client for any reasonable cause. Reasonable cause includes a client asking you to do something that goes against what you believe is right or that your professional code of ethics states is inappropriate. If your professional code does not clearly state a boundary issue, you should confidently stay committed to your own beliefs and values about what is right and wrong.

SCENARIO

Your client has referred her sister to you because of the sister's high-stress job. Both sisters continue to see you weekly on different days. While receiving a massage one day, your original client asks how her sister is doing. You tell her she is doing well. She begins to pry for more information, asking if you know why her sister is so stressed. She also asks how long her sister's sessions are and how often she comes to see you. She seems truly concerned about her sister.

1. Can you give your client the information she is asking for? _____
_____

2. What should you say to your client regarding treatment of her sister? _____
_____

3. Is there any part of a professional code of ethics that can help you decide what to say to this client? _____
_____

In the scenario presented, the client's questions lead the therapist to review her policies and codes. The original client was most likely genuinely concerned about her sister. Explaining the guidelines for confidentiality in your code of ethics would assure the sister that you must keep all information about all clients confidential, even among family members. If a situation arises when you feel a session is not in compliance with your ethical standards or professional code of ethics or if a client is placing you in an unsafe situation, you have the right to stop the session and ask the client to leave. You also have the right not to schedule any further appointments with the client. The safety of both the therapist and client is an important ethical issue. If a client does something that may be against a law or regulation, it is important to end the session. This issue is discussed more fully in Chapter 4 on laws and regulations.

Key Points

- Know your ethical boundaries.
- Practice how to tell a client about your ethical code.
- Clients can make innocent requests, not knowing they are asking you to break your code.

APPLYING CODES OF ETHICS IN YOUR PRACTICE

Even before you graduate and begin your practice in bodywork, you should embrace a code of ethics for your profession. While still in school, begin practicing the ethical standards and following the guidelines that you will use throughout your career. Give every massage to fellow students the same as if the student were a client. This will help you practice and begin to feel more comfortable when working on actual clients. If you practice in a student clinic, you will likely experience clients asking questions that may put you on the spot, and you may be unsure how to answer. Look to your instructors, supervisors, or mentors to help you know how to answer such questions or requests. Practice talking to clients and answering questions with your fellow students. Addressing requests and answering questions confidently help assure clients that you have strong convictions in your ethics.

Once you begin to practice, like many practitioners you may choose to be affiliated with a group or association that has a code of ethics. Many massage therapists display a copy of this code of ethics in their office for their clientele to see, and some may include the code in a brochure or flyer given to clients. Not all clients take the time to read the entire document, but they may still notice that you follow a code of ethics. A client who still has some reservations about massage or bodywork may be reassured by reading that you follow a specific code of ethics.

Therapist can also write their own expanded version of a code of ethics. Based on your personal values and beliefs, you may feel the need to clarify certain issues or even add areas that are not covered in other codes. Many individuals work in facilities where more than one therapist practices, sometimes with a staff having a number of different backgrounds, such as in physical or occupational therapy. In such cases a client could easily be confused and ask you to perform services you are not trained to do. Educating the public and other facility personnel helps them understand that it is your ethical responsibility to work within your scope of practice.

SUMMARY

Even the best codes of ethics and standards cannot address all the possible issues that a practitioner may encounter while doing bodywork. Clients have various physical and emotional issues you should be prepared to handle. Issues involving trauma, abuse, physical handicaps, and body functions can all present dilemmas for bodyworkers. Many of these issues are addressed in later chapters of this book, and you can discuss them with other students and instructors. Such discussions can introduce you to situations that you may not have thought about when you chose this profession. As you encounter such issues, you will see the importance of understanding and having tools such as a code of ethics to help handle difficult situations. As you read the following chapters, keep your beliefs and values in mind. You now have the foundation for your own personal code of ethics, and by the end of this book you will be ready to write your own ethical code.

LAWS, RULES, AND REGULATIONS

4

CHAPTER PREVIEW

- Laws, rules, and regulations affecting your massage therapy business and your actions
- Why and how laws are made
- Importance of knowing laws, rules, and regulations
- Ethical practice within the boundaries of laws, rules, and regulations

KEY TERMS

Accountability: showing the responsibility or proof of performing a task or duty

Civil law: system of law involving relationships or disputes between two parties

Criminal law: system of law regarding actions that are harmful to the public

Laws: rules established and enforced by governing bodies that protect or restrict actions by all citizens or specific parties

Ordinances: rules and regulations established at the local level

Regulations: rules of conduct that are often associated with laws, involving an expansion or explanation of the laws

In almost every walk of life, laws, rules, and regulations affect how we act. Laws, ranging from guidelines for duties such as paying taxes to protecting us from injury, violence, and damage to our personal belongings, affect everyone. Laws and regulations are rules that governing bodies have determined people must follow. In most cases the governing body also states the consequences for people who do not obey the laws.

Laws are enacted not only to protect the public from harm but also to keep agencies and governing bodies running smoothly and with **accountability.** With civil law, for example, governing bodies give citizens the right to file a lawsuit against another party for damages when they feel they have been wronged.

In this chapter, you will learn about the importance of laws, rules, and regulations; how they affect your massage practice; and how ethical behavior involves working within laws and regulations.

LAWS

Laws are passed to protect the public, to keep governing bodies running effectively, and to set guidelines for appropriate behavior. Almost all countries have some structure of laws that states what behaviors are acceptable and what are not. The laws of different countries vary greatly, often depending on the type of government that runs the country and that society's ideas of right and wrong. In the United States we elect officials at the national, state, and local levels to set our guidelines. Literally thousands of laws, rules, and regulations are created every year by these governing bodies.

Each level of government establishes rules of conduct for a defined population. Our national governing body is the U.S. Congress, the legislature, a branch of the federal government. We elect representatives and senators to serve in Congress. They create the laws for the entire nation for matters such as taxes, the environment, criminal acts, and business operations. Federal laws and regulations apply to everyone in the United States.

At the state level, we also elect officials who serve in a state legislature. The laws and regulations created by this body affect people living only within that state. A state legislature passes laws, for example, that may give the people in that state additional protections beyond those in federal law. A state cannot pass a law that is contradictory to a federal law, however. For example, if the U.S. Congress passes a law making it illegal to dump certain chemicals in any river, a state cannot override that law to authorize this dumping in the state. In some instances, the federal government may set certain general guidelines for the entire nation but allow states to determine specific aspects of that regulation. Setting the speed limits for highways is an example. The maximum speed limit may be 65 or 70 miles an hour for all federal highways, but a state can set a lower speed limit in areas it deems dangerous. Other areas are left entirely to the states to determine what laws may be needed. This is the case with licensure for massage therapy. Currently some states have laws and regulations pertaining to massage, while in other states only cities or counties have regulations. Some areas have no state laws or regulations or local ordinances that apply to massage therapy.

Currently, no national laws govern the practice of massage and bodywork. Although it might seem beneficial to have consistent laws, rules, and regulations that apply to all therapists in all locations, there is no present movement toward this goal. The National Certification Exam is currently accepted as a test for licensure in many states, but it is not required at the national level. Not all states that require licensure for massage and bodywork accept the National Certification Exam as a requirement for their state licensure. Because of such differences, you must research the laws and regulations of any state or area where you are thinking of building a practice.

THE RELATIONSHIP OF LAW AND ETHICS

Laws and ethics are closely related but are not the same thing. Many laws are based on ethical principles. For example, it is unethical to hurt someone, and laws also make this a criminal act and apply some form of punishment.

When a law is broken, police and the court system take action against the offender. With a civil offense, individuals may file lawsuits against others who they feel have wronged them. When an ethical offense occurs, however, it may be a professional association that takes action against the offender. For example, if a client feels unfairly treated by a therapist, the client can file a complaint with the association, which then determines if indeed an unethical act has occurred and what should be done.

Laws at the national and local levels cover many actions and behaviors, but they cannot cover every possible aspect of what is right and wrong. Unscrupulous people will always try to "bend" the law or find loopholes in the law. A society's ethical principles may clearly indicate what is right or wrong, but unfortunately some individuals will not behave within those parameters but may still avoid breaking the law.

The law also changes to reflect current beliefs and issues. For example, in the early and mid-2000s, our society has emphasized business law and ethics. Many criminal and civil proceedings involved corporations and their owners or directors. Many criminal cases and individual lawsuits focused on activities involving the stock market. In general, laws change with the times and a society's needs. Ethical principles, however, do not change as easily, because our society generally has a strong foundation of right and wrong. Yet at times ethics and the law may conflict. For example, some would argue that legal limitations on gay rights in some areas conflict with the general ethical principle of fairness.

Massage therapists should accept the responsibility to know both the laws and ethical codes that apply to their profession. This information is readily accessible with research. Even if you do not join a professional association, adopting an accepting ethical code for your own professional practice will help your clients know that their well-being is important to you.

WHO MAKES LAWS?

Laws, **ordinances,** rules, and **regulations** are all created at various levels of government. Citizens must follow all federal and state laws as well as local ordinances. State laws generally have similarities and differences from state to state. For the practice of massage and bodywork, 33 states now have some regulations. Most of these states define criteria for a license to practice, such as a certain number of hours of massage training, and many require a certification examination. In addition, most create a board to oversee practice and the profession within the state. In other states, local or county regulations often apply to therapists. It is the responsibility of all therapists to become educated about what local, county, and state regulations apply to their practice.

States differ, however, in other regulatory matters, such as the number of hours of training required, the type of examination used, the makeup of the board that regulates the profession, and the cost of licensure. For example, in some states the medical board oversees massage practice, while other states have a separate board that regulates only massage.

Often local ordinances also regulate the practice of massage. Some community ordinances have education requirements for therapists, some require background checks and health examinations, and some regulate geographical areas where a practice can or cannot be located. Some communities have no specific regulations at all for massage and bodywork businesses. Most communities have general regulations that require anyone opening any business to have a business license. Some communities have additional rules and regulations for certain types of business such as massage therapy, doctor's offices, manufacturing plants, and food establishments. Every therapist planning to work in any community should ask at city hall or the county offices about the requirements for practice within that community. Opening a practice without completing the proper paperwork could lead to closure or fines by the local authorities.

Therefore, you need to know all laws and regulate pertaining to your location. You will learn your own state's requirements during your massage training, but if you are considering practicing in another state, you should contact officials there to learn its requirements for massage practice. Among different states, the training requirements range from 300 to more than 1,000 hours of training in order to be licensed to practice massage and bodywork. When relocating, you should contact both the state and local governments about licensure requirements. For example, if your current school offers a training program of 720 hours and you are thinking about relocating to another state, you should first contact that state's secretary of state office to learn how many hours of training are required. If it requires more than 720 hours, you will need additional training before you can begin practice there. Many other professions such as nursing, chiropractic, athletic training, and physical therapy are also regulated by state guidelines and laws.

PROCESS OF MAKING LAWS

In the United States, at the national level, the government has three primary branches: the legislative, executive, and judicial branches. Congress is the legislative branch that, in keeping with the Constitution, passes legislation for laws and regulations. Congress consists of senators and representatives elected to serve in the Congress. The executive branch also consists of elected officials, led and directed by the President. The judicial branch consists of the federal

court system, in which federal judges are appointed by the executive branch and confirmed by the legislative branch. The Constitution designed this system of checks and balances to prevent any one branch of government from having too much power. For example, the executive branch can veto a law made by the legislature, and a court can rule on the constitutionality of a law. All branches are subject to the principles of the Constitution.

In general, laws are created because a need is shown for some type of regulation. Interested parties, agencies, or legislators assert that some regulation is needed for a particular behavior or practice or for the regulation of a professional group. For example, health care for elderly individuals is a major concern in our country today. Many legislators are looking at ways to make health care more affordable for elderly people. Many states are considering laws to reduce the cost of prescriptions, medical treatments, and nursing care. Special interest groups representing the elderly population present their arguments to a state legislator who may then propose a bill with specific steps to protect the group. Legislators may also reject the arguments of special interest groups proposing legislation if they do not believe there is a need for the new legislation or do not believe the legislation could pass. Different states have enacted laws regulating massage for a variety of reasons. Some view such laws as a way to protect the public from unscrupulous practitioners, while others may do so to provide guidelines for the education of massage therapists and to define the scope of practice for massage therapy.

Once a senator or representative decides to propose a new law, the process begins. The proposed legislation, called a bill, is first written. In most cases, this step requires study and research and possibly many months of writing and rewriting. Different interested parties often work together during this process to produce a final version of the bill, which is then presented to the legislature. In the case of massage practice, interested parties may include national and state massage associations, coalitions, special interest groups, and individual therapists. It is a costly process to produce legislation, and in many cases the funding is supplied by one of these groups. Special interest groups, associations, and coalitions help with this process to assure that laws and regulations are written to help ensure the safety of the public and to ensure that therapists are not unfairly restricted in their practice. For example, testing massage therapists for sexually transmitted diseases would be not only unrealistic and unfair but a burden for many.

The next step is for the legislature to consider the bill. The bill is introduced, is given a number, and is usually referred to a committee. A bill concerning massage and bodywork may be referred to a professional licensing and regulation committee or to a health care committee; each state has its own system of committees. When the committee receives a bill, it has three choices. It can set up hearings, discuss it within the committee, or decide not to discuss it at all. The committee chair often makes the decision whether a bill does or does not move forward.

Another group or individual can affect the legislative process at this point: lobbyists. A lobbyist employed by an interested party or business meets with the committee chair or other legislators to convince them of the need for passing the bill. At the same time, a lobbyist from another group opposed to the bill may be trying to convince the committee to drop the bill. Lobbyists can be hired by any group with an interest in the outcome of the legislation. Associations, coalitions, businesses, and special interest groups often fund the proposed legislation and lobbyists. Massage associations too have worked with lobbyists to affect the outcomes of legislation.

While the committee is considering a bill, it may hold hearings. In a public hearing anyone with an interest in the bill can make a presentation to the committee to argue for or against the bill. In addition, if committee members see a need for a change in the bill, they may rewrite a portion of the bill.

Once the bill is final, if the committee decides to bring it to the full Senate or House of Representatives, the bill then passes to that legislative body for discussion and a vote. At this stage the media often report on legislative debates about bills that involve some controversy. If the bill passes the first legislative body, it then goes to the other body. For example, a bill that passes in the House of Representatives then goes to the Senate for consideration. In the Senate it is assigned to another committee, which goes through the same process again. Often the full process from proposal to enactment of a law can take 3 to 5 years. In any given year, most state legislatures consider 100 to 200 bills. This process involves a considerable amount of information, especially since most state legislatures meet only 3 or 4 months of the year.

If changes are made to the bill while it is in the second house, it may be sent to a committee made up of legislators from both houses, called a conference or consensus committee. This committee tries to work out the differences, and if they do, the revised bill is then sent back to both houses for a vote. Lobbyists are often involved in all aspects of trying to get the bill passed.

Once a bill passes through both chambers without additional changes, it then goes to the governor to be signed into law. The governor has the right to veto the bill if he or she disagrees with it. The legislature then may or may not attempt to override the veto with another vote. If the governor signs the bill or the legislature overrides a veto, the bill becomes law.

Listed below are some examples of laws governing massage therapy:

- The state of Missouri requires a minimum of 500 hours of massage training in a state-approved school. This includes instructors who have been approved by the State Board of Therapeutic Massage.
- Florida law states a license can be denied or disciplinary action can be taken for fraudulent representation in the practice of massage.
- Some states now require all massage therapists to have continuing education hours for license renewal.

On the local city or county level, governing bodies establish regulations, generally called ordinances. An ordinance adds to existing federal and state laws to meet the specific needs of the community. For example, a business license is required in most communities. Local ordinances may also require a building inspection, business applications, and a business fee to open a business.

Elected officials at the local level may be called city councilors, aldermen, or selectmen. They perform in much the same way as legislative officials do at the state and national levels. An interested party who sees a need for guidelines brings a proposal before the city council or board. The board may consider the proposal or may refer it to a special group or committee for a recommendation. Public hearings may be held to hear the community's opinions, followed by further debate or a vote.

Local requirements for massage therapists, like state regulations, can be quite diverse. In some communities, old ordinances and regulations can hamper massage therapists today. Many of these ordinances were enacted to restrict massage parlors. For example, in some cities it is illegal to operate a massage business within 500 feet of a school, church, or bar. Many massage therapists have worked to help update such outdated regulations.

Listed below are some examples of local ordinances that still affect massage and bodywork:

- Any person engaged in the practice of massage must submit to a background check for a criminal record.
- A person wishing to practice massage within the city limits must undergo a health examination by a licensed doctor.
- A massage therapy practice must keep a log of all clients for a minimum of 2 years.

EXERCISE 4-1

Contact two therapists in your area and ask if you can interview them. Ask questions such as these:

1. What state laws and local ordinances affect you and your practice?

2. Were these laws in place when you opened your practice or did they come about after you were already in business? If the latter, what changes did you have to make?

3. Have these rules affected your practice in a positive way?

4. Have these rules affected your practice in any negative way?

5. Should additional rules be made to protect you or your clients?

Report back to your class what you have found.

■ A window must be present in any massage room.
■ A person wanting to practice massage must undergo a check for sexually transmitted diseases.

ENFORCEMENT OF LAWS

Once a law is passed and is on the books, that law must be enforced. The law itself specifies who is to enforce it. For example, **criminal laws** are enforced by the police and court system, which act upon violations of that law. People who break the law are arrested and brought before a court to determine if they are guilty or innocent and what the appropriate punishment should be.

In cases such as the regulation of a profession, a state board may oversee enforcement of the law. A state board is usually made up of people in the profession, who work to help therapists follow state laws and regulations and who respond to violations. For example, if a bodyworker is practicing without a required state license, the board may send a cease-and-desist order stating the person must stop the practice of bodywork until he or she has applied and been accepted for licensure. If this person does not stop practicing, he or she could be subject to a fine or other penalty, again according to what the law prescribes. The law or regulations related to it generally define what the board has the power to do when a violation takes place.

All professional boards must work within the requirements of the laws. If a law states a board can fine a person for practicing without a license, the board can do so upon evidence that this violation has happened. Boards work with legal council, often a state attorney, when enforcing laws and regulations. A practitioner who has questions or concerns about a law should always address the state board for clarification.

Key Points
■ Most laws are made to protect the public.
■ Currently, laws, rules, and regulations affecting massage and bodywork are passed and enforced at the state and local levels.
■ Laws, rules, and regulations vary at the state, county, and local levels.
■ It is important to know what rules apply to you in your practice.

CASE STUDY

Judith had graduated from massage school about a year ago and had been working at a local spa several days a week. Then because of her husband's job relocation, they had to move to another town a few hours away. Since massage therapists can move fairly easily, Judith was confident that she could start another practice in their new town. After moving, she looked for a good location for her practice. She decided to open her own office and have space for other therapists to work.

She checked with the city offices to obtain copies of any rules or ordinances that applied. She had found a great location and was getting anxious to get a lease signed and open for business. She read the ordinances and found that a massage practice could not be located within 500 feet of a church, school, or bar. The ordinance seemed rather archaic to her, and as it happened, the office space she wanted to use was close to a small church. When she called city hall and inquired about this, she was told this ordinance had been on the books for over 25 years and would be enforced.

Judith contacted one of the alderman in her town and asked about the possibility of changing the ordinance. The alderman listened to her arguments and asked her to state her case at an aldermanic meeting. She was put on the agenda for the next meeting. Judith did some research, including contacting the national association that she belonged to. The association provided her with information about why these ordinances had originally been passed and how many communities had changed or updated such rules. Judith appeared before the board and presented a valid case for changing these rules. The board agreed with her and thanked her for her education about massage therapy. This rule was then changed, and Judith opened her practice a month later.

RULES AND REGULATIONS

When a new law is enacted, the governing body may set up a state board to oversee the law. In many states, the board is appointed by the governor. The board generally has 5 to 10 members, most from the profession involved, but many states also appoint a member of the public or someone from a related field. For example, some states may require that a nurse or chiropractor sit on the state board of massage.

The board's goal is to make the law work in practical ways for the profession. This requires a set of rules and regulations, often called the "rules and regs." The rules and regulations expand on the law itself, including explanations for how practitioners should do what the law requires. The board cannot go beyond what the law states it should do, and in most cases one of the state's attorneys helps the board determine where this line is. Typically, once a law has passed and the board is seated, it can take more than a year to write the rules and regulations. Checks and balances are important, and in most states once the rules are written, a public hearing is held to allow practitioners and the general public to respond to the proposed rules. After the public hearing, the board may rewrite the rules and regulations as needed to work more efficiently.

Rules and regulations are important to help delineate the law. Most laws involve general principles and contain general language that may seem vague in certain areas. If laws were left to individual interpretation, opinions would vary about what they mean. Rules and regulations, therefore, help define the intent of the law. For example, a law may generally state that massage therapists must practice the principles of safe sanitation, and the rules may more specifically state that a 10% bleach solution must be used to disinfect all equipment that comes in contact with clients and that massage therapists must wash their hands with an antibacterial soap between clients. As simple as this may sound, it is important for the rules and regulations to be clear and specific guidelines so that there is no room for varying interpretations. For example, if a client complained that a therapist did not use good sanitation, unless the rules and regulations clearly defined good sanitation, the board could have difficulty determining whether the

therapist was sanitary or not. Clearly defined rules can prevent varying interpretations of the law.

Another example is a clarification of the exact amount of training needed for licensure. The law may state that 500 hours of training are required. The rules may further state that certain numbers of hours are required in certain categories such as anatomy, physiology, kinesiology, massage theory and techniques, pathology, ethics, health and safety issues, and cardiopulmonary resuscitation.

WHY RULES AND REGULATIONS ARE NECESSARY

Rules and regulations are extensions of the law intended to guide those affected by the law in practical applications. The rules and regulations help to guide persons in the specifics of what is acceptable and unacceptable in their practice. It may take a long time and considerable effort to change a law, but a rule or regulation that is not working can generally be changed with less effort.

More importantly, the rules are there for those whom they affect. They protect both the public and the therapist from harm with clear-cut guidelines. For example, if a client files a complaint against a therapist about insufficient draping and the state regulations clearly define what the minimal draping should be, the state board can then work with the therapist to use draping practices that are appropriate for clients. If the regulations did not clarify the specifics of required draping, however, board members would then have to determine what they felt was appropriate—an issue that, again, is subject to a great deal of interpretation. Rules and regulations are necessary to reduce the amount of interpretation needed to determine whether a violation has occurred.

From an ethical viewpoint, rules and regulations can help prevent ethical questions and situations from arising in the first place. With the draping example, some therapists may not see it as an ethical issue if a client is not draped, yet the client may feel violated. But if a regulation states that certain areas of the body must be covered during massage, then the rule is very clear. If a therapist ignores this rule, the client has cause to file a complaint. Regulations are also helpful in the opposite case. If a client does not want to be draped, it is easy for the therapist to tell the client that not using draping is against the state law.

Another example is a regulation that requires the client's informed consent for treatment. Some states specifically state what information is required for massage treatments. An additional example is a requirement of confidentiality for all clients.

A new state law was enacted, and the state board began writing rules and regulations for a public hearing. This state law defined massage. Chair massage was not specifically mentioned in the law or the regulations, and some therapists assumed that licensure was not required if they performed only chair massage. The state board heard about this interpretation and decided to revise the regulations to include language regarding chair massage to clarify that therapists who performed only chair massage were also affected by the law.

It is important not to interpret laws, rules, and regulations on your own. When in doubt, ask your governing body.

ENFORCEMENT AND CONSEQUENCES

Laws specify who oversees enforcement and the consequences of violations. When a criminal act is committed, for example, law enforcement agencies are directly involved with arresting suspects and pressing charges. A trial and possible sentence may follow. If a regulatory law is violated, the state board accepts a complaint, holds a hearing, and makes its determination. If a therapist is found at fault, the law or the rules and regulations provide the board with enforcement guidelines. For example, if a therapist performs a technique not within his or her defined scope of practice according to state law, a client could file a complaint with the state board. Following the rules and regulations, the board would then determine what action to take against the therapist. Actions could include a letter of reprimand, or suspension or revocation of a therapist's license to practice.

CIVIL LAW

Civil law is another type of law governing people's behavior. In a lawsuit, one party feels that he or she has been harmed in some way by another party. There may not have been a clear violation of a law or regulation, but the person could still be harmed. Rules and laws address as many issues as possible, but there can be gaps that allow for civil actions to take place. Unethical behavior may be involved. In civil law, one party (called the plaintiff) files suit against another party (called the defendant), seeking damages or restitution. For example, a client may feel a therapist has injured him or her in some way during a therapy session, causing pain and suffering. If the client feels the therapist caused this injury, the client may seek financial damages from the therapist.

In civil cases law enforcement agencies and the state board may not be involved. Instead, both parties are represented by lawyers. The case may end with an out-of-court settlement, or the parties may go to court to settle their differences. If so, a judge or jury weighs the arguments of both sides and reaches a decision about whether the defendant did in fact cause an injury and the amount of damages to award the plaintiff.

In reality, anyone can file a lawsuit against anyone else at almost any time. Being sued does not mean you are guilty of anything, nor does a lawsuit automatically lead to any penalty. The legal system is set up to protect the innocent as well as to provide compensation for injured parties. **If you practice massage therapy as you have been trained and within your scope of practice, you should not be afraid of lawsuits.**

Key Points
- Rules and regulations define areas of the law.
- Rules and regulations clarify the practical specifics of laws.
- Rules and regulations provide guidelines for both therapists and the public.

SPECIFIC LEGAL ISSUES

SCOPE OF PRACTICE

The scope of practice for a massage therapist can be defined by a state law, professional association, or local ordinances. The scope states what a therapist can or cannot do while practicing as a massage therapist, technician, or bodyworker. These parameters help therapists understand what the public expects from massage therapy and, more importantly, states the boundaries for therapists. For example, a state law may include in the scope of practice that a therapist can use certain mechanical devices.

Scope of practice can vary somewhat between a state's law and a professional association's statement of scope. Although they may be very similar in many ways, therapists must be aware of any differences and must practice under the definition enforced by state law. It is important therefore to read and understand your state's scope of practice regulations.

MALPRACTICE INSURANCE

Malpractice insurance is a type of insurance for professionals that pays the damages a professional may face if sued by a client. Medical malpractice lawsuits are often in the news, and most medical professionals purchase malpractice insurance. Medical malpractice premiums are generally expensive because lawsuits are common and juries often award large sums for damages. In massage therapy, few lawsuits are filed against therapists are low, and malpractice insurance premiums. Malpractice insurance can be purchased through professional associations or a private insurance broker. One should do some research to choose the best and most appropriate policy. Several insurance companies offer policies specifically for massage therapists and bodyworkers. Some states now require massage therapists to purchase malpractice insurance.

CONTRACTS

Massage therapists enter into contracts with employers, employees, clients, landlords, insurance companies, and other businesses, depending on the type of practice. For example, therapists working in a spa may have a contract with the spa that spells out the expectations for both parties. In many situations only a verbal agreement takes place between the two parties.

A contract is a legal document, and as a general rule it is good to seek legal advice before signing any contract. Both parties should agree on all terms of a contract. If someone pushes you to sign a contract, such as an employment contract if you are hired by a facility, do not be intimidated to sign without reading the document. Thoroughly read the entire contract and have someone else help you determine if the contract is fair before signing. If needed, changes can be made to help both parties come to an agreement.

SPECIFIC ELEMENTS WITHIN LAWS

State laws may include a great variety of specific legal issues. When you are preparing to become licensed or to practice in an area, obtain copies of laws, rules, regulations, and ordinances pertaining to your practice. Many therapists are surprised to discover how many details are contained within these documents. A state law may address client confidentiality, for example, or issues such as employer liability and responsibilities. Do HIPAA **(Health Insurance Portability and Accountability Act)** regulations referring to client records apply in the state? Could certain antidiscrimination regulations affect a massage practice? If you have any questions concerning any part of a law or ordinance, contact the governing body and don't be afraid to ask questions. Understanding the expectations before beginning practice is much better than having to make changes later when a problem arises because you did not know about a specific regulation or ordinance.

Laws and regulations do not apply only to those who run their own business. Even if you practice within someone else's business, the state laws and local ordinances still apply. For example, if you work in the office of a chiropractor, you are not exempt from laws and ordinances within your area. Being informed and educated about the law is all part of being a professional.

THE IMPORTANCE OF BEING IN THE KNOW

When you decided to begin a career as a bodyworker, you took on the responsibility of learning how to practice appropriately. This involves not only being well trained in massage techniques but also knowing the expectations of governing bodies. "I didn't know" is not a legal defense—and is not an excuse that any professional should ever use. Both the general public and those who enforce the law expect you to know the laws that apply to your practice.

Before you begin your practice, it is crucial for you to learn about any laws, rules, regulations, and ordinances that may pertain to your practice. You may need to check at the national, state, and local levels. If your state requires that you take the National Certification Examination, for example,

EXERCISE 4-2

1. Obtain a copy of your state's law regulating massage therapy. If your state does not currently have a law, research whether legislation is currently in process. Using the Internet, look for the Web site of your state government. Most state sites allow a search using key words for proposed and passed legislation. Obtain a copy of any legislation or laws that will apply to you and your massage therapy practice. Note: If you do not have access to a computer, you can also call the secretary of state's office, which should be able to guide you to the appropriate department or documentation.

2. Go to city hall in the city where you think you may establish a practice. State that you will soon be graduating from massage therapy school and want information about local ordinances that apply to practice. Obtain copies of any local ordinances or regulations along with a business application.

3. Show and tell. Tell classmates what you have learned about your state's and community's requirements.

and a local ordinance states that you must have 750 hours of training in order to practice, you cannot practice until you meet both of these criteria. Most massage programs teach their students at least the state-level requirements. It may be up to you, however, to learn what is expected at the local level. Take the time to get all the specifics—it's better to be safe than sorry. There have been cases of therapists who set up a practice only to find out they did not meet the requirements in their local community.

Therapists should also stay networked within the massage community to stay current in the law. Laws, rules, and regulations change sometimes, and such changes can affect how you practice or your whole career. For example, if your state increases the number of continuing education hours required for license renewal, you would need to make plans to meet this requirement.

CASE STUDY

A therapist who had been in practice at a hospital for a number of years decided to venture out on her own. She found a great office location in a community where no other therapists were practicing and rented the space. She had to put down a sizable deposit as this was a very good neighborhood and available spaces were hard to find. She bought furniture and hired a receptionist and had 5,000 brochures printed along with cards, gift certificates, and stationery with her new address. She put an ad in the paper for her grand opening, which cost her more than $1,000. She was excited about her new place of business and her grand opening.

Then she got a call from City Hall asking when she was going to apply for her business license. The city clerk had seen her ad and knew she had not processed an application. She immediately went to City Hall, thinking she would probably have to pay $100 and fill out some paperwork (Fig. 4-1). When she arrived, she found that the city required a building and fire inspection, which would take about 2 weeks to complete. Her grand opening was already set for the following week. The city clerk tried to help her meet her deadline, but the fire inspector found a couple of code violations and the building inspector also found some problems. The landlord was willing to make the fire inspector's changes, but the building inspector was asking for more changes than the landlord felt he could afford from the rental income generated by her space. The former tenant had run a one-person private office and did not meet with the public. Her public business would require the landlord to add two extra parking spaces and handicapped access into the office. In the end, the therapist had to forfeit a great deal of money, because her lease stated that the landlord did not have to make improvements and that deposits would be forfeited if she left before the lease expired.

This mistake was a hard lesson for this therapist to learn, but is a valuable one for all therapists to hear. If the therapist had first checked with city hall and had the inspections before putting a deposit on the office space and spending money on printing and advertising, she could have saved a great deal of time and money.

It is the responsibility of all massage therapists to become educated in legal matters and understand what laws, rules, regulations, and ordinances apply to them (Fig. 4-2). **It is also important to not interpret any laws, rules, and regulations on your own.** When in doubt, ask the people in charge. Talk to your state board or your city government. Students sometimes feel frustrated in having to deal with officials, but this is part of the educational process and there is much to be said for knowing just what you have to do. The Internet is often a valuable resource for getting information and applications when needed. In addition, check with your school and other therapists in your community to see what they have done, but be careful when acting on personal information because not

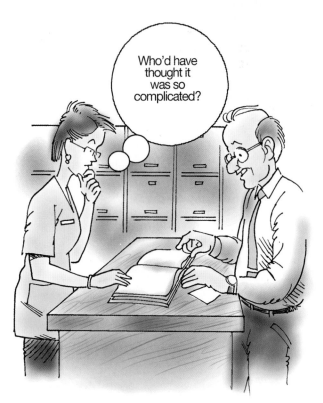

FIGURE 4-1 ■ A new therapist should research local ordinances that apply to her business.

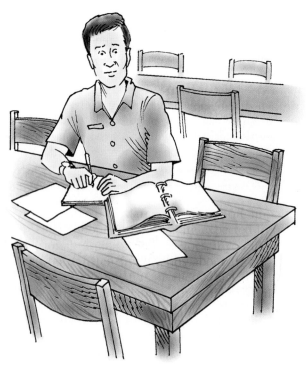

FIGURE 4-2 ■ It is the responsibility of all therapists to know what laws, rules, regulations, and ordinances apply to their practice.

everyone follows all the appropriate guidelines. When in doubt, ask. If you are the first therapist in your community, don't be surprised if your city officials are unsure about appropriate guidelines for massage therapists. In this case, you may need to meet with the officials to help create guidelines for your community. Find ordinances and regulations from other communities to help the process along. Be patient, and remember the person you are talking to may become a client or someone who tells other people about your new practice.

Key Points

- Know your state and local regulations and laws.
- Not knowing is not an excuse.
- Research and ask questions.

SUMMARY

Knowing the legal requirements for practicing as a massage therapist or bodyworker makes it much easier to attain that goal. State laws and local ordinances will likely affect your practice, and it is your responsibility to know what these are.

Laws, rules, regulations, and ordinances may seem overwhelming at first, but realize that they are there for your protection as well as the public's protection. During your career as a therapist, at times a law or a rule will provide safety and helpful guidelines for dealing with a difficult situation or client. Laws and rules help to define many areas, but a therapist must also take the responsibility to act ethically when the rules leave room for interpretation. In some cases old rules or ordinances on the books may seem irrelevant, archaic, or old-fashioned. Be proactive and help educate those who can help update these rules. Being aware, setting your boundaries, and knowing the importance of acting ethically will be a tremendous boost for you as a therapist and for your clients as well as the general public who may become clients in the future.

ADDITIONAL ACTIVITIES

After you and your classmates have a sense of what laws and rules apply to a massage therapy practice in your area, have a class discussion to answer these questions:

1. What areas of the law or rules protect clients?
2. What areas of the law protect therapists?
3. Do any areas of law restrict the practice of massage or cause hardship for therapists?
4. Do any areas of law need more definition?
5. How many of the therapists you and your classmates interviewed were well educated about laws and regulations?
6. How would you go about changing a law or rule that needs revision?

5

BOUNDARIES

CHAPTER PREVIEW

- The importance of boundaries for both the client and the therapist
- Why boundaries are sometimes crossed
- Defining and maintaining boundaries
- How to manage a crossed boundary

KEY TERMS

Boundaries: limits between acceptable and unacceptable behaviors

Emotional boundaries: limits for keeping therapeutic sessions focused on the client's body rather than emotions

Physical boundaries: the physical lines or limitations in relation to a client's body that a therapist should not cross

Professional boundaries: the limits of acceptable professional behavior

Sexual boundaries: limits to prevent ever sexualizing any aspect of bodywork

Social boundaries: limits for keeping the relationship with clients professional rather than social

Boundaries are one of the most important dimensions of the practice of massage therapy and bodywork. Issues involving boundaries are among the most frequently discussed topics by professionals in practice and are also often an area of concern for new and potential clients.

What exactly are boundaries? The word itself is often used in two different ways. First, there are personal boundaries between you and the client: **physical boundaries, emotional boundaries,** and so on. If you have ever been unexpectedly touched by a stranger in a public place, you know what it feels like to have someone cross your personal boundary. Obviously, massage therapy involves touch, but there are still boundaries between the therapist and clients in terms of where the body is touched and how.

A second meaning of the word boundaries involves limits of behavior. We often speak of "crossing the

line" or "going too far" when issues of acceptable or unacceptable behavior are involved. In this sense the boundary is the limit, the line between acceptable and unacceptable. Often in massage therapy both meanings of boundaries are present at the same time. For example, a boundary issue occurs if a therapist touches a client in a sexual way, because the therapist has crossed a boundary between self and the client and has also crossed the line from acceptable behavior to unacceptable behavior.

Laws, rules, and regulations define many necessary boundaries, such as **sexual boundaries** and physical boundaries. In other areas, however, boundaries are not always so clear-cut, and there is no simple set of rules that everyone in the profession follows. New and even experienced practitioners can have difficulty defining and understanding where exactly the boundaries are. It is often challenging for new practitioners to know exactly where lines need to be drawn. The standards of the profession leave some things open to interpretation about what is acceptable or unacceptable for both the therapist and clients, sometimes causing confusion. It is not always clear what guidelines should be followed.

In the therapeutic relationship, a therapist also cannot always know precisely what the client may view as acceptable or unacceptable. How can you know if you are crossing a line if a client does not bring it to your attention? Establishing your own general guidelines and discussing and defining them individually with each of your clients would seem to take a great deal of energy and time. Nonetheless, you can start your career with a strong foundation of your own principles, knowing where your boundaries are and accepting the guidelines of the profession. This chapter explores why boundaries are important for both the therapist and clients, what happens when lines are crossed, and how to manage boundary issues in your new practice.

THE IMPORTANCE OF BOUNDARIES

There are several different types of boundaries in the therapist–client relationship. These include physical boundaries involving issues such as draping, what areas of the body should or should not be worked on, and the types of work performed. Emotional boundaries between the client and therapist are also important. As Elliott Greene and Barbara Goodrich-Dunn write in *The Psychology of the Body,* "Boundaries of behavior serve to facilitate the therapeutic process, create safety, and protect the integrity of the client and therapist." The therapist and client should agree where the appropriate boundaries lie in the bodywork relationship. From the time you enter into a professional relationship with a new client, the client should expect you to maintain the parameters of that relationship.

Yet all too often, the professional relationship can begin without clear definitions of the parameters or boundaries that both parties feel are acceptable. To help prevent this potential problem, some therapists include a brief section on their intake form that states their scope of practice, and other therapists ask new clients to read their written policies before sessions begin. In these ways therapists can describe their boundaries for clients. But clients, too, come into the professional relationship with their own expectations regarding physical and professional boundaries, and it is similarly important for the therapist to know what these

expectations are in order to work effectively with the client. The therapist and client both need to communicate their expectations and parameters to each other to begin a productive therapeutic relationship.

DEFINING BOUNDARIES

Boundaries are based on guidelines that help you maintain a professional image for your clients and others in the profession. Establishing and maintaining your own exact boundaries is an important step in the practice of bodywork. Still, most therapists eventually face unanticipated situations or situations in which the usual rules do not seem to apply. In situations like this, you may need to be somewhat flexible while remaining strong within your beliefs and foundation. For example, if a state regulation states that clients should be provided privacy while dressing and undressing but a disabled client needs assistance undressing, the therapist will need to still maintain as much privacy as possible for the client while assisting.

BOX 5-1   *Types of Boundaries*

Physical boundaries involve physical limits that neither the therapist nor client should cross. In some states, laws, rules, and regulations spell out clear-cut boundaries in this arena. Where there are no rules to follow regarding physical boundaries, clients generally expect the therapist to have guidelines that help them feel safe..

Example: When you are working on a client's inner thigh, the draping creates a line that a therapist should not cross. A client who feels unsafe or unsure about you working in this area may react by saying something or showing discomfort by tensing up, moving away from your hands, or fidgeting on the table. Even though the sheet is the physical boundary, a client can still feel uncomfortable while the therapist works on different parts of the body.

Social boundaries are boundaries between a therapist and client that prevent the relationship from becoming too social rather than professional, including the expectations by each that the other will follow acceptable standards of behavior.

Example: A client enters into the therapeutic relationship expecting to receive services from you. The client does not expect you to make the sessions a socializing experience to form a social relationship. But if you were to talk continually about your personal life or feelings during the client's sessions, as you might with a friend, you would have crossed the social boundary line. This can also happen with a client trying to make the therapeutic session a social event.

Emotional boundaries involve limits between the therapist and client related to emotional issues or problems. Therapists should focus on working on the client's body, for example, rather than trying to address emotional problems a client may seem to have. Although there certainly is an emotional component of bodywork, most clients do not expect to become emotionally involved during the massage session. Clients mostly think of the physical relief that they will feel at the end of a session. Even clients who are aware of their emotional response after receiving a massage do not expect a therapist to provide counseling to address this aspect of their lives.

Example: You may easily cross an emotional line when a client exhibits an emotional response to bodywork you are doing. It is natural to try to nurture your clients, but stepping over the line and trying to address issues usually considered in the realm of counseling or psychotherapy is dangerous for both you and the client and is beyond your scope of practice.

Sexual boundaries are limits that prevent sexualizing bodywork. These limits are generally defined in laws and regulations. Massage therapy professionals all agree that massage and bodywork must not be sexual in nature.

Example: Sexual boundaries include more than the obvious transgressions involving sexual behavior. A therapist whose thoughts or emotions become sexually oriented during a session, going beyond the purely therapeutic aspects of massage, is crossing a boundary line. If while working on a client you begin to feel an attraction to the person, your touch will likely change and the client may notice that something else has entered the relationship. This can also happen if the client is attracted to the therapist. In either case, problems are inevitable.

Professional boundaries involve guidelines and expectations related to professional behavior. Governing bodies, associations, and peers have definite expectations for what the therapeutic relationship should be. The laws of many states specifically define the scope of practice for massage therapists. Many laws also state what a therapist cannot do. Some practice areas are clearly defined, although others may leave room for individual interpretation.

Example: Clients frequently look to massage therapists for advice on a wide range of health issues. For example, clients may ask you what vitamins they should take. Unless you are specifically trained in nutrition, you would be crossing a professional line if you gave advice in this area. Many clients also confuse chiropractic therapy and massage therapy, and may ask you to perform spinal manipulation. This would also be crossing a professional boundary unless you are also licensed as a chiropractor.

When working with the public, you need to be aware of all types of boundaries. In some cases you may have to find a balance between your own professional expectations and the expectations of an individual client. Finding a middle ground requires thought and practice. For example, a client may not feel comfortable removing any of their undergarments, which can be challenging to work around in certain areas such as the back. Explaining any limitations this may have during the session will help the client understand the work being done and the boundary issues involved. Knowing when a client is deliberately or unconsciously testing the boundaries of your relationship is also often important in maintaining a successful practice. You cannot expect all clients to know where all boundary lines lie. Most clients assume that you, as a professional, know where the lines are and will keep them in a safe therapeutic relationship.

On the other hand, most therapists have other clients who do not know the boundaries and may consciously or unconsciously challenge the limits. It can be a challenge to keep the professional relationship intact in such cases, as in the common situation described in the scenario.

SCENARIO

You are shopping for groceries on Saturday and encounter one of your clients in the checkout line. Unfortunately, the store is busy and you both have to wait a few minutes in line. Looking into your grocery cart, the client casually says that it looks like you are having a barbecue and asks if you are having a party. You say you are just having a few friends over, but she continues to ask questions about where you live and other aspects of your personal life.

1. Would this situation make you feel uncomfortable?
2. What would you say to this client?
3. How can you maintain a professional relationship without appearing cold to this client by refusing to answer her questions?

It is not possible to be prepared for all possible client situations that you may encounter in your professional career, but the better you understand the different boundaries you need to maintain, the more clearly you will know when lines are being crossed and what to do about it. If you begin to feel uncomfortable in a situation with a client, boundary issues may be at the root of the problem. It is then important for you to assess what, if any, action to take or not take to preserve the therapeutic relationship.

SCENARIO

You are performing bodywork on a client who has been a wonderful client for several years. She is always happy and upbeat, and your sessions always end on a happy but professional note. During this session, however, she mentions that she is having a party and would love for you to come. You have a professional policy against socializing with your clients. You try to change the subject gracefully to avoid having to tell her no, but she keeps talking about it and insisting that you should come to her party.

1. How would this make you feel?
2. What would you say to this client?
3. How do you maintain the therapeutic relationship in this situation?

Key Points

■ Boundaries help set parameters for your practice.
■ Boundaries help assure your clients they are in a safe environment.
■ Some boundaries may be defined by laws, rules, or regulations.
■ When boundaries are not clearly defined by laws or a governing body or association, therapists should define their own.

Your personal boundaries are directly related to your values and beliefs, as discussed in Chapter 2. The strength of your commitment to your boundaries may also depend on your past experiences. Before beginning Exercise 5-1, you may want to look back at what you wrote in the Chapter 2 exercises.

Professional boundaries are generally defined by associations, groups, laws, and rules. For example,

EXERCISE 5-1

List two boundary principles in each of the four areas that you feel strongly about.

Example: Physical boundaries: I feel all clients should disrobe only as far as they are comfortable.

Physical boundaries:

1.

2.

Social boundaries:

1.

2.

Emotional boundaries:

1.

2.

Sexual boundaries:

1.

2.

many association codes of ethics state that practitioners must work only within their scope of practice. Scope of practice is defined by several massage associations as well as many state laws. These documents also help the public know the professional expectations for practitioners. In your own practice area, if you find aspects of practice you feel are not covered well, you can formulate your own additional policies to address those areas. If you do not agree with the established boundaries, you may need to look for other practice options, such as joining a different professional association, moving to a different state, and so on.

BOUNDARIES FOR THE THERAPIST

As you prepare to enter practice in the massage and bodywork profession, you should consider your comfort and professional boundaries when working with clients. In an earlier chapter you explored how your personal belief system evolved and what your beliefs and values are today. These beliefs and values form a foundation for your guidelines related to boundaries with clients. At the same time you have seen that your fellow students have many diverse beliefs. Likewise, your clients will bring their own beliefs, values, and boundary issues to the professional relationship.

It is important to know where your boundaries lie and what to do when they are questioned or crossed. Therapists who enter practice without thinking through these issues can get into trouble because of unclear parameters when working with clients. Or the client may feel or sense that the therapist is not steadfast and therefore feel uneasy during the session.

CASE STUDY

Cindy was looking forward to a massage session she had booked with a new massage therapist in town. Her previous therapist had moved away recently, and Cindy really liked receiving a massage every other week to reduce stress. Her previous therapist had been in business for 8 years and always kept her sessions very professional, always addressing the areas Cindy wanted worked on.

The new therapist gave Cindy a good massage, but she also spent much of the massage telling her about her personal problems. Her car wouldn't start that morning, and her boyfriend had been a total jerk, and she just wanted to go home and have a nice dinner.

Cindy felt good physically after the massage, but she was not as relaxed as she usually was in the past because of all the therapist's talk during the massage. When she left she did not book another massage and was unsure if she would ever come back to this therapist because of all the chatter.

In a situation such as Cindy experienced, the therapist had not set effective boundaries to prevent inappropriate behavior or conversation with the client. Social boundaries that restrict sharing personal information are an important component in any therapeutic setting. Is the client paying for a massage session that includes hearing your personal problems or other personal information? Unfortunately, it is a common complaint among clients that their massage therapist spent most of the session talking about all sorts of things, when all the client wanted to do is relax.

Boundaries are also needed for the techniques you perform. Through your career as a bodyworker, you will learn new techniques and skills to enhance your sessions with clients. Your clients expect you to perform all techniques with expertise and not use them to practice skills you have not yet mastered. It can be a difficult situation when you have just learned a new technique but are still not very good at it, yet you want your clients to benefit from this technique. In such a case, it is generally better to practice on a family member or another therapist until you have mastered the skill.

SCENARIO

Bill recently attended a weekend class in craniosacral work, an area in which he has been interested since he graduated from massage school last year. This was the first in a series of classes, and he planned to attend others as his budget allowed. He learned a great deal of information during the lecture portion of the class, but because of the size of the class he had only a few hours of hands-on time with these new techniques. He had told several of his clients that he was taking this course, and the next week several clients asked him to use the new techniques on them.

1. Should Bill practice these new techniques on his clients?
2. Should Bill tell them he has not had much practice yet, but will spend a few moments using the new techniques?

3. Should Bill charge them for this new service?
4. Should Bill practice only on other therapists and family members until he becomes proficient in the new techniques?

Deciding when to practice new techniques on clients is a subjective issue. Especially when you are a new therapist, it is difficult to be sure when your skills are good enough to use on paying clients. Following are a few suggestions to help you determine what is best for your clients and yourself:

1. Ask the person who taught you the skills when he or she thinks you can begin to use them on regular clients.
2. Check to see if a set or standard number of hours or series of classes is normally required in this technique. Your instructor may suggest a minimum number of hours of practice before using a new technique on clients.
3. Check to see if any certifications or examinations are used to determine proficiency in a new technique or skill.
4. Research and practice new techniques until you feel you know a great deal about them.

Another type of boundary, which is very clear-cut in most codes of ethics and state laws, is the rule against sexual contact or any sexualizing of massage. Some members of the public still associate massage with prostitution, and even all the regulations against sexual behavior do not convince these people. This boundary issue arises if a client requests something beyond this boundary. Many therapists have reported that, at some time in their career, a client either came right out and asked or subtly hinted at wanting the therapist to cross over this boundary. Having clear-cut boundaries helps you out of this situation, and the client will understand that you have a strong foundation.

EXERCISE 5-2

This exercise is a personal journal exploring where you are today.

1. I know I will never _____ with a client.

2. I know I will always _____ with a client.

3. I think I will never _____ with a client.

4. I think I will always _____ with a client.

Try to expand on your thoughts and write a sentence or a paragraph for each of the items above.

CASE STUDY

A therapist who has been in business for 2 years repeatedly had clients try to overstep her boundaries against any form of sexual relationship. On average, at least one client a month hinted about wanting to take her out and have an intimate relationship with her. Finally she had enough and asked one of her teachers at her massage school for advice. After talking for awhile about these clients and asking questions about how the sessions went, the teacher asked her what she wore to work every day. The therapist said she dressed for work much like she was dressed today. She was wearing tight black pants and a low-cut top that was somewhat revealing. The teacher explained that her clothing might be interpreted by some as suggestive, somewhat as some bar waitresses dress to attract good tips. The teacher suggested that she wear more professional attire for her practice in the spa setting. After trying the different clothing for a month, this therapist found that clients had all but stopped approaching her in inappropriate ways.

A therapist's boundaries are even more important than clients' boundaries. You are expected to be the professional. As an old saying goes, if you like something you will tell five friends about it, but if you hate it you will tell ten. If clients feel you do not have a strong foundation, they may think your practice is not ethical—and they may say that to many others.

Your boundaries help keep both you and your clients safe. Maintaining clear-cut boundaries also lets the public and potential future clients see that you are serious about your business and maintaining a professional practice.

BOUNDARIES FOR THE CLIENT

A client may cross a boundary with a request or behavior that is innocent or that the client knows is inappropriate. Your job as a professional is to handle both situations in an appropriate and business-like manner. Ideally, you should be prepared to handle almost any situation that may present itself.

An example of an innocent request is a client asking for advice on nutrition or to be shown strengthening exercises, when you are not trained in these areas. Many clients believe that bodyworkers are trained in all aspects of the body. They may not understand the difference, for example, between a massage therapist and a physical therapist. Simply explaining to your clients that this kind of advice or work is beyond your scope of practice should help them understand that you are not trained in this area. Clients who persist with such questions may be referred to another health care professional.

In situations in which a client deliberately and inappropriately crosses a boundary, being prepared can help you handle the situation in a professional way. Learning to say no in a professional yet firm way is an important skill to manage a client who asks you to cross a boundary. The professional way to address this situation is to explain that the requested action or information is not within your scope of practice or

---

EXERCISE 5-3

Practicing how to talk to a client who makes an inappropriate request should be an important part of your training.

Pair up with another student. One is the therapist and the other the client. Use props as needed (desk and chair, massage table, massage chair). Different pairs of students use the following scenarios. Take the time to compose your scenario and present it to the class. Afterwards, the rest of the class should offer suggestions for how to handle the incident.

1. A new client calls to make an appointment for a massage. He asks a lot of questions including what the therapist will be wearing.

2. A female client tells her male therapist that she would like to have lunch with him sometime soon.

3. A male client asks his female therapist for advice about a problem in his marriage. He keeps bringing it up during the session.

4. A male client does not like to be draped and keeps taking the draping off during the session.

5. A female client breaks down and starts crying while the therapist is working on her back. She seems to have experienced an emotional release and tells the therapist she has been abused.

6. The therapist has been working with both a husband and wife. Now the wife asks a lot of questions about her husband, including what he talks about during sessions.

Try to avoid the temptation to turn these scenarios into humorous situations. It is important to practice what you may have to say to a client in situations like these when asked to overstep a boundary.

---

would violate state laws, regulations, or your own practice policies. If the client persists, you need to end the session—or never make the appointment in the first place if the client requests it in advance. You have the right to refuse to treat a client for just and reasonable cause.

If you are unsure how to cope with a client crossing boundaries in your practice, and you want to keep this client, it is appropriate to consult with a mentor or ask a teacher for advice. Often another person can see the situation more clearly from a different viewpoint and can help dispel the emotional response often evoked by situations involving boundary issues.

> **Key Points**
>
> ■ Clients generally expect a therapist to have set boundaries.
> ■ Clients are less likely to try to test your boundaries if they know you are a professional committed to maintaining your boundaries.
> ■ Believe in your boundaries. Clients will feel your firm commitment to your profession.
> ■ Be prepared for instances of intentional or unintentional boundary crossing by clients.

CONSENSUS BETWEEN THE THERAPIST AND CLIENT

It is important for a therapist and client to reach an understanding of each other's expectations for the therapeutic relationship. Each party begins this relationship with expectations, and unless they communicate to each other their expectations, it may be more difficult for this relationship to be successful. Effective communication should begin with the first phone call to make an appointment and should continue throughout each session.

When a potential client calls to make an appointment, that person is in a sense checking you out to see if you will give the treatment he or she is seeking. The person also wants to feel safe. If you say anything that makes the person feel uncomfortable, he or she may not make the appointment or may not show up for the appointment. For example, if a potential client asks what clothing is worn during the session and the therapist simply answers that the standard policy is to remove all clothes, this could make the person feel very uncomfortable. A better answer would be that clients are encouraged to disrobe only as much as they are comfortable and that draping is used throughout the session to keep them feeling safe and comfortable. If the potential client still hesitates, the therapist can then explain what happens during the massage session and ask if the person has any concerns. It is important to listen carefully to the client to learn what concerns and issues may be present. In the example above, the fact that the client asked about clothing suggests the client could be uncomfortable with disrobing, and a therapist who is listening carefully will take note of this and respond appropriately.

During the intake process, try to identify any fears or concerns that a client may have. Often these issues are very subtle, and if you are not paying close attention to what the client is saying and how the client is responding, you may miss the cues. Pay attention to questions that clients ask

---

| BOX 5-2 | *A Conversation With a Prospective New Client* |

Since you are new in business, every new phone call may make you nervous. It is important to be professional and maintain your boundaries from the very beginning. The call might begin like this:

Therapist: Thank you for calling The Massage Connection.
Client: Yes, I'd like to know what types of massage you offer and the prices.
Therapist: Well, we offer several types of massage. Our techniques include Swedish, sports, reiki, aromatherapy, hand and foot reflexology, and Thai massage. The prices vary from $65 to $90 per hour.
Client: Which one is best for relaxation?
Therapist: For general relaxation, many clients like Swedish massage or aromatherapy massage.
Client: What would I wear during the massage?
Therapist: Well, you take off your clothes and we have sheets for you.
Client: You mean I have to take off everything?
Therapist: Yes, we usually don't have any problems with that.
Client: Well, I'll have to call you back.

Observe where this client begins to feel apprehensive about what the therapist is saying. The first call is a time to engage your client and listen for concerns. When you hear the client begin to sound nervous or question something you have said, take action to make the client feel more comfortable.

At the point where the client asks what he or she will wear, the therapist could better have proceeded like this:

Client: What would I wear during the massage?
Therapist: Your comfort level during your massage is very important to us. During the session, you will be fully draped with only the area that we are working on uncovered. We respect your privacy and ask that you undress only as much as you are comfortable. We use sheets and towels to cover you during your massage. If you have any concerns, we'll talk about them before your session.

In this case, as the person begins to trust the therapist and the session, the new client may more readily feel at ease and not get nervous removing clothing for the session.

---

and to their body language. If clients still seem to have concerns after you have answered their questions with full explanations, ask them if they still have concerns. Be gentle and open in your conversation. It is important to watch and listen to a person's reactions during conversations at the beginning of the therapeutic process and relationship. You must provide a safe ground for the relationship to become established and build.

Although this verbal communication is very important, the physical communication that occurs during a session is one of the most important aspects of bodywork. You are being trained to receive messages from your client's physical body so that you can most effectively treat the body. These physical messages tell you about are problems such as adhesions, spasms, triggers points, and scar tissue. Clients may or may not be aware of such problems. Likewise, clients may not realize that their bodies are reacting physically to emotions and feelings from the past or that they feel now during the bodywork session. For example, if a client has an area of injury from a minor fall, you may find some adhesions or restrictions in that area that can be effectively treated by different forms of bodywork. But if that minor fall was associated with some type of emotional pain, the client's emotional reaction may be much more significant than the physical trauma. A client may tense up or even cry while you are working on an area, but probing the client in an effort to discover what is causing the emotional response would be crossing a boundary outside the scope of practice of bodywork. At such times communication, understanding, and nurturing the relationship can be very critical. Working within your scope of practice, you help clients within their comfort level and work toward the healing process as bodyworkers are trained to do. Pushing clients to explore their emotional or personal response is not within your scope of practice.

Clients may not feel comfortable discussing an issue with you that may be revealed during a bodywork session. For example, while you are working on a client's shoulder, you feel the client tensing up and pulling away from you while you work. You should check the client's pressure and pain levels to make sure that you are not hurting the client. If the client says that the pressure is fine and the pain not significant, there could be an emotional reason why the client is responding in this manner. The client may not even realize that it is happening. Asking clients if they feel any discomfort is appropriate, but it would not be appropriate to ask more questions in depth about why they seem to be responding emotionally. Sometimes a client goes home and thinks about what happened, and may tell you about the injury or event during the next session or two. Another client may never want to talk about such issues at all. Still other clients will open up and tell you everything and want you to solve their emotional problems. Working within your scope of practice and professional boundaries is very important in situations like this. It may also be important to refer such clients to other health care professionals to assist them in the healing process. If a client seeks help for emotional trauma, it may be appropriate to refer the client to a counselor, psychologist, or psychiatrist. Explaining to the client that this is beyond your scope of practice helps the client know why you cannot offer advice in this

area and that you have the client's best interests at heart to promote healing.

Verbal and nonverbal communication should be an ongoing process with all your clients. Communication needs are unique for each client and every session. It is important to stay open to changes that can happen and know that your boundaries will keep your professional relationship safe.

Key Points
- Two forms of communication take place with any client during therapy sessions: verbal and physical.
- Verbal communication is the conversation that you and client have before, during, and after a session.
- Physical communication involves energy that is exchanged between a client and a therapist. It is crucial for a therapist to be aware of this during a session because this information can be critical for the care of the client.

HOW BOUNDARIES ARE CROSSED

Clients and therapists can cross boundaries in a variety of ways. It may happen unintentionally, such as when a client does not understand your scope of practice. It can also be intentional, such as therapists going beyond their scope of practice and performing techniques or procedures they have not been trained to do. Because the practice of massage and bodywork is so diverse in this country, it is important to know your scope of practice within any rules, regulations, laws, and guidelines applicable to your practice.

CROSSING A BOUNDARY WITH TOUCH

As discussed earlier, all clients come into the therapeutic relationship with their own expectations and possibly even apprehensions about what will happen during the session. A new client may have had massage sessions with another therapist and may expect you to follow a similar format. Other clients may have never received any type of bodywork and do not know what to expect other than they want to feel psychologically and physically safe during the session.

This can be a delicate topic to discuss with new clients, but it can be handled professionally through the intake process. Your intake form can ask what areas of their body they do or do not want worked on. Some intake forms have boxes listing all parts of the body, and clients simply check what they feel comfortable having worked on. Without use of such intake information, it can be difficult to discuss this openly with a new client during the initial interview. Nonetheless, it is important for your clients to know that their feelings of safety are important during the session and that if anything concerns them at any time, they should feel free to speak up.

As you train in the bodywork profession, you naturally let go of some of your own inhibitions as you realize the need to work on parts of the body that some people are sensitive about. For example, most new therapists at first have difficulty addressing the gluteal region, but when you see the positive effects of work in this area, it seems only natural that this part of the body in many cases needs work. Your clients may not feel the same way, however, and have not had time to address the issue. If you do not have permission to work here and you undrape the area, the client may not feel comfortable with work in this area. Sometimes you need to take a more conservative approach and slowly educate the client about work on sensitive parts of the body. Clients should have the choice to allow you to work on sensitive parts when they feel ready. Clients may give you blanket permission for bodywork when they come to you, but it is important for you as a professional to ensure they always feel safe with what you are doing. Forcing clients to accept something they feel uncomfortable with can be very intimidating and is not taking care of the client. If they do not feel safe and their needs are not being met, they may not return. In the worst possible scenario, a client who feels he or she has been touched inappropriately may file a complaint with a state regulating agency, local authorities, or other entities such as an association in which you are a member. Verbal and physical communication can help prevent this situation from happening.

A client too may cross a touch boundary. A client might touch the therapist in a way that is not appropriate for the therapeutic relationship. This can be very surprising when it happens, in which case it is important to consider whether it was purposefully done. Talking with the client and explaining that the act was inappropriate will help the client understand the importance of your boundaries. You may need to be careful with this client in the future, and if the client persists in acting inappropriately, you may need to end the therapeutic relationship.

CASE STUDY

A female therapist has worked on a male client weekly for the past 2 years. He has repeatedly come close to pushing personal issues, such as by asking her if she has a boyfriend or what she was planning for the weekend. On several occasions the therapist reminded him what her professional parameters were. He then backed off and made no advances for a while. Now, however, during a session while in the prone position, when the therapist was working on his shoulder from the side of the table, he grabbed her leg and made a playful comment about how smooth it was. The therapist stopped her work and told him that this type of touching was not appropriate. He commented that a little innocent grab did not hurt anyone. The therapist then stopped the session and told him that they were done for the day. Even though he then apologized, the therapist felt it was important for this client to get the message that he had crossed an important boundary. When he asked about his next appointment, she stated that they would not be having any future sessions. The therapist felt she could no longer maintain the professional relationship and took control by ending their work together.

Even though a professional relationship is a joint venture between two parties, it is important to understand that you have the responsibility for setting important parameters for your safety and the client's safety. Clients who are truly interested in a therapeutic relationship will understand that boundaries should not be crossed.

CROSSING A BOUNDARY WITH WORDS

How and what you say during your career as a bodyworker can have a profound effect on your success. You have likely noticed how people take interest when you are talking about your new career as a bodyworker. Many people are keenly interested in this field and want to understand more about it. That is in part why it is important to choose your words carefully when talking about massage so that friends, family, and potential clients see that you work with professional parameters.

Remember that some people still feel massage involves some sort of sexual overtones. Some students of bodywork react with anger when hearing such comments, while others say nothing at all. It may be better to consider this an opportunity to educate someone who has the mistaken impression that massage is wrong or unsavory. Talk to the person in a calm and effective way. Avoid becoming defensive, and find a way to guide the person to a new thought process. What you say can have a tremendous effect on what people think. Learning how to approach people with a variety of different ideas is an important skill in our profession.

A therapist had been working on a client for the last several months. During the last session he mentioned to this client that she really had a great tan. The client thanked him for the compliment. He then asked if she was tan all over—in other words, did she tan in the nude. This question could certainly make the client feel uneasy. Commenting on the tan may be okay, and being concerned about the risk for skin cancer is certainly important to anyone interested in health. The client could have accepted comments from that point of view but likely began to feel uneasy about discussing tanning in the nude.

Inappropriate conversation during a session can also become an important issue in a therapeutic relationship. Clients expect you to be the expert and often look to you for advice. **Always think about what you are saying to a client and be careful to stay within your scope of practice.** Giving advice on topics in which you have not been trained is inappropriate. Even simple things like telling a joke may be inappropriate if the client may misinterpret it or find the joke offensive. A joke involving any aspect of sexuality may make a client feel uncomfortable. Always consider what you are saying before you say it, and be responsible to maintain the therapeutic relationship.

There are many boundaries that we must be aware of when working with the human body. Comments about body types or parts can offend someone very easily. Stay aware of what you are saying and how you phrase information to your clients to ensure that they are not offended or hurt by what you say. For example, rather than saying to a client who is overweight, "It is hard to work through fat," it is more appropriate to refer to working in "areas where there is more tissue."

Although it seems like you are always having to think about what you say and what you do, many of these aspects will become natural as you gain more experience in the bodywork field. Awareness of the responsibilities and the consequences is an important part of your training now.

CROSSING A BOUNDARY WITH NONVERBAL COMMUNICATION

Nonverbal communication scares many but is discussed by few. It can cause more problems than many other issues discussed so far. Nonverbal communication may involve a simple look, smile, or even touch that is intended or perceived differently by the therapist and the client.

Clients look to their therapist for relief from pain or stress. Most clients really like and appreciate their therapist and look forward to their sessions. But if a therapist smiles at a client or gives a casual hug, the client may feel the therapist is flirting. A client may see more meaning in something as innocent as a smile if the client is looking for the therapeutic relationship to provide more than it should. Therapists need to be aware of the power differential with clients (discussed in the next chapter) and understand why it is important never to take advantage of that type of behavior.

Another potential problem is touching the client in a way that the client may perceive as something other than a massage technique. Clients receive the therapeutic effects of massage, but allowing the massage to mean something else is dangerous. For example, if you feel a client is very good looking and you are thinking about that during the massage session, your thoughts can influence how you touch the client, who may then feel that the massage is taking on a more seductive feel. Massage and bodywork involve an energy exchange between two people, and energy from your thoughts too can be transferred to another person. Consider the different ways clients can feel your touch while you are giving a massage. Clients can feel your emotional state, such as anger, complacency, impatience, sexual attraction, or love. Therefore, your frame of mind during the session is just as important as the skill in your hands.

FLEXIBILITY OF BOUNDARIES

Many boundary issues involve solid rules that should be followed in the bodywork profession. As you have seen in the ethical codes of professional associations, some behaviors such as sexualizing massage are clearly viewed as wrong. But in certain aspects of the therapist–client relationship, such as the social arena, you can be somewhat more flexible in your practice. Your behavior in this respect may depend on the individual client. Adapting to each client can be challenging for a new therapist, but you can do this without much stress or thought. For example, many clients would like you to be personable rather than always strictly businesslike in your relationship. Some clients may want to tell you about their kids or an upcoming special occasion that is affecting their stress levels. When you see clients regularly, it is good to show an interest in their lives. But when the social aspect of the relationship starts taking time or energy away from the sessions, it becomes necessary to draw a line. It is not difficult to casually step back into the therapeutic role by simply saying that you need to focus on what is going on physically with the client's body. Clients sometimes lose track of the purpose of the therapeutic relationship and may just like the fact that someone is listening to them. Remembering that it is your responsibility to make the therapeutic relationship work for both of you, find a comfortable way to do your work so that clients leave the session feeling their needs have been met (Fig. 5-1).

With some clients you may need to be stricter with social barriers because the client is unable to distinguish between a social and therapeutic relationship. You usually know when this happens because you begin to feel frustrated or uneasy in the sessions. If you lose your focus on the session and the work you are doing, this is a sign that the therapeutic relationship is at risk. Refocus the client on the work that you are doing by asking appropriate questions about his or her reaction to the massage. If a client persists with social comments or questions, simply saying something like "Let's concentrate on this shoulder right now" or "Tell me what you are doing at work that causes your lower back to hurt" is a way to let the client know that you are

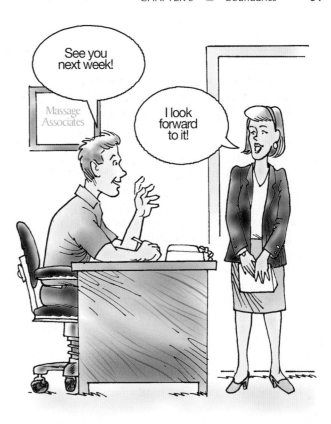

FIGURE 5-2 ■ It is possible to have a pleasant, personable relationship with clients while remaining professional.

trying to focus on your work. If the client still persists, you may have to be more direct and say that you need to focus your attention on the session.

Flexibility with your clients allows you to have a professional yet personable relationship. It is a very good feeling when your clients feel right at home with the sessions and leave feeling better both physically and mentally (Fig. 5-2).

MANAGING CROSSED BOUNDARIES

Maintaining boundaries in the bodywork profession is a continually evolving process. You could not easily write a clear-cut document defining what all your parameters will always be. Yet you know your own expectations at the present.

Because you already have a belief and value system in place, you have a good sense of what your practice parameters will be. As you complete your education and gain more experience in the field, you will continue to develop those parameters in a comfortable fit for you and your clients.

Regardless of your own sense of boundaries, however, clients may unintentionally cross a boundary and you may have to decide how best to handle the situation. For example, a client may tell you a joke

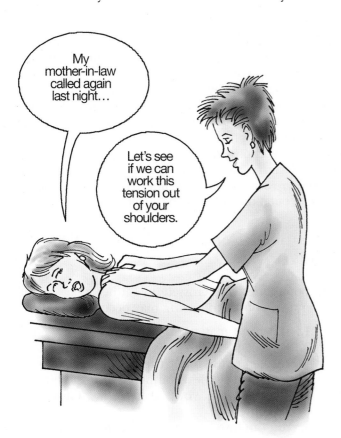

FIGURE 5-1 ■ You may have to help clients focus on issues related to the massage rather than their social or emotional life.

about religion. The client may think there is nothing wrong with the joke, but you may find it offensive. Is it appropriate to say something to the client and risk making the client feel bad about telling the joke, or is it better just to let it go? You may face such boundary issues almost daily, and that is why it is important to understand your own foundation. A therapist should weigh the client's potential response if you tell the client the joke offended you. Sometimes it is more appropriate to let something like this go, unless the client continues with offensive remarks or jokes. In this case, telling the client that this type of conversation is offensive may be appropriate. Another example is a client who unintentionally lets a drape fall off and does not realize what has happened. Adjusting the sheet would be the appropriate action. If the client constantly lets the sheet fall off, you may need to say something about staying covered during the session.

CASE STUDY

A new client has come to you for some work on a sore back. You take the client through your normal intake process and explain how the session will proceed. You ask the client to lie on the table in the prone (face down) position under the sheet. When you enter the room, the client is lying face up with no sheet. What would you do?

A simple solution is to exit the room and ask the client to please turn over and get under the sheet. The client may have been nervous and unsure about positioning on the table.

Clients may also ask you to step outside your scope of practice. This usually happens because they do not know the exact scope of practice for bodyworkers. They also may not understand the nature of your training. A brief explanation of the types of work you do would be helpful during the intake and interview process and allow the client to ask questions about things they may not understand. Some clients may think we have the same training as physical therapists or chiropractors and that we can perform the same techniques. One example that is quite prevalent is a client asking a massage therapist to perform a spinal manipulation. This is usually a chiropractic technique that is outside the scope of practice of massage therapists. Simply telling the client that this technique is outside your scope of practice is usually enough, or if not, just say you are not trained in this area. These boundary issues do not involve repercussions when handled in a professional manner.

Some clients intentionally ask you to cross boundaries. First, explain to the client what your boundaries are. If the client persists and continues to ask you to step outside your boundaries, you have the right and responsibility to end the session or no longer see this person as a client.

CASE STUDY

Tanya had a client who had come for two massage sessions appointments in two weeks. During his third session he began to ask a lot of personal questions. He asked if she was married or seeing someone. Tanya explained that she did not discuss her personal life. He quieted for awhile but then said he noticed that she was not wearing a ring, so he just wanted to know what her boyfriend thought of her working on men not wearing clothing. She again stated that her personal life would not be discussed during the session and that if he kept pursuing this, she would have to end the session.

Near the end of the massage the client told Tanya that he found her very attractive and wanted to take her out. Tanya decided that it was best to end the session early, and told the client she would see him in the outer office when he was dressed. When he came out, Tanya told him that it was against her policy to date clients and that he should seek another therapist for future sessions.

Whenever you face a situation like Tanya's, you have to choose whether to terminate the therapeutic relationship with a client. Often clients will understand that you have boundaries that you will not cross, and once you have explained this, they will stop asking you to cross those boundaries. If a client continues to push, you can end the session and, if necessary, choose not to see that client in the future. These can be hard decisions to make, but once you have crossed a boundary line, your self-confidence and reputation will likely be affected.

WHAT CAN HAPPEN IF BOUNDARIES ARE CROSSED

If boundaries are crossed by either you or the client, any of the following may occur.

1. The client may not return.
2. The client's needs may not be met.
3. You can refuse to see the client again.
4. A client may file a complaint against you.
5. You can lose your license (in states with licensure).
6. You can lose membership in an association.
7. You may gain the reputation of not being an ethical practitioner.

None of these options is a good experience for a bodywork practitioner. Somewhere along the way, someone is going to lose. The cost can be as simple as losing a client or as high as losing your career. Because the stakes can be so high, it is important to address boundary issues continually in your practice.

Key Points

■ Boundaries may be crossed by the therapist or client through touch, words, or nonverbal communication.

■ Some boundaries are absolute and not open to interpretation, whereas others are more flexible depending on your relationship with a client.

■ If a client intentionally or unintentionally crosses a boundary or asks you to do so, you must manage the situation before a problem results.

Paying attention to your client's needs while providing a quality, ethical service will help clients see you are a professional. A strong foundation and preparation to address any problem that arises are the tools to handle any situation that you may face.

SUMMARY

As you worked through this chapter, you have learned how to address more of the issues that you will face in your bodywork career. At first, it may seem there are many different issues to prepare for, but it really comes down to basics. Acting ethically should be a part of who you are and what you do. Knowing your boundaries and having a strong foundation will help you every day in your practice. Clients will know and feel that you have their best interests in mind and will provide them with an ethical service. Clients need to feel safe, and respecting boundaries helps provide this safety. Communicating with and educating your clients are continual processes that will evolve as you gain years of experience. But if a problem arises, do not hesitate to consult a mentor to help you through a tough situation.

CLIENT AND THERAPIST RELATIONSHIPS

6

CHAPTER PREVIEW

- Understanding the dynamics of the power differential in a therapeutic relationship
- Managing the transference of thoughts and feelings from the client to the therapist and from the therapist to the client
- Problematic and successful dual relationships

KEY TERMS

Countertransference: a therapist attributing thoughts or feelings about another person to the client

Defense mechanisms: behaviors that unconsciously protect a person from feelings or awareness

Dual relationship: a situation that occurs when two roles or relationships overlap or interact

Power differential: the shift of authority that can exist in the client–therapist relationship

Transference: a client attributing thoughts or feelings about another person to the therapist

---

The dynamics of the relationship between and therapist and client can be diverse and complex, and attending to these is just as important as the techniques used during a bodywork session. Successful bodyworkers pay close attention not only to the techniques that they use but also to the many details involved in the relationship with clients. Marketing, physical client comforts, music, and follow-up are all important business aspects a therapist must pay attention to, but more important is the nature of the relationship that you form with your clients. Ethical issues play an important part of this relationship, and the therapist should maintain a constant awareness of this relationship. Variables involved in this relationship are discussed in this chapter along with suggestions to help make sometimes challenging situations workable for both parties.

POWER DIFFERENTIAL

A client who seeks you out as a massage therapist does so because he or she believes that you have had training in your field and are considered reliable to provide the services desired. Clients want to trust that professionals know what they are doing and look to them to provide a quality service. For example, when you take a ring to a jewelry store to be fixed, you assume that the jeweler knows how to fix the ring correctly. But what guarantees do you have that your ring will be fixed properly? You simply assume that this person has the power or ability to fix it. The same holds true when you see a doctor or dentist, or have someone fix your plumbing or work on your car. Our society assigns this power to professionals, and in turn many professionals act upon this power because it is the expectation of their clients. This power develops from a psychological expectation in many cases rather than from actual facts. For example, many clients assume that a bodyworker can evaluate their range of motion. A bodyworker can assess that there is a problem, but a full evaluation of the nature and degree of the malfunction in most cases is beyond the scope of practice for bodyworkers.

The client's assumption gives a therapist a great deal of power, psychologically trusting that the therapist will know what type of work should be done. Clients believe and trust that they will receive the service the therapist has promised. When you ask a mechanic what is wrong with your car, you most likely will believe what he or she says and trust that what is wrong will be fixed. In other words, we grant that the mechanic has the power to fix the car and we do not. Likewise, your clients look to you for professional advice about what you think is wrong with them and trust that you will provide a therapy that will be helpful to them.

A client takes on the role of being cared for in a therapeutic relationship. For example, when you see a doctor because you do not feel good, you are seeking the doctor's advice and treatment. The doctor will diagnose your condition and possibly provide a medication or other treatment to help you get better. You accept that the doctor has the power to take care of you and help you get better. A client who receives bodywork also assumes the therapist has power to determine what is wrong and provide an appropriate type of treatment in order to feel better. Relative to the professional who provides the treatment, clients feel "powerless" to treat themselves. This powerlessness is an important component of a therapeutic relationship. The difference between the professional's power and the client's powerlessness is called the **power differential** in the therapeutic relationship. A responsible therapist is consciously aware of the dynamics that can happen with this power differential and takes care not to take advantage of the client.

HOW THE POWER DIFFERENTIAL AFFECTS CLIENTS

Clients look to you as the professional who understands bodywork and should know everything about techniques and their problems. It is very common for clients to look to you for advice regarding what you think is wrong with them. They essentially are asking you to diagnose what ails them. Most state laws and many ethical codes state, however, that massage therapists and bodyworkers do not diagnose any type of disease, symptoms, or maladies of clients. Yet clients often ask bodyworkers for their opinion and seek some idea as to what is wrong with them. This can be a very difficult situation for a new therapist in two ways. First, you most likely do not know enough about medical conditions to understand fully the cause of their symptoms. Many symptoms can be caused by any number of problems, and figuring out what their disease is or the cause of their problems requires more training than bodyworkers receive. Second, it can be difficult to explain to a new client that you cannot diagnose health conditions. Therapists really do want to help, but explaining to your client that diagnosing any type of medical condition is beyond your scope of practice is the best thing to do.

The power differential has many dimensions in addition to expectations about disease and symptoms. Clients may also look to you as someone that they can confide in or someone who can soothe their emotional pain. You are working on tissues with a great deal of memory, and doing bodywork can bring other psychological or emotional issues to the surface. Clients may then look to you to help soothe their feelings or just listen to what they have to say. This in itself adds an immense amount of responsibility to the therapist's role in the therapeutic relationship.

As the therapeutic relationship develops over time, a therapist will understand more fully why a client wants to receive massage, why the client has pain, and how the client deals with problems and pain. It is much like fitting together the pieces of a puzzle to form a picture that makes sense. The client looks to the therapist to understand what is happening to his or her body and use therapeutic skills to make it better. Clients come for a massage with a purpose and give the therapist the power to make them feel better. Some clients may simply need relaxation, while others need pain relief, corrected posture, or simply a positive touch. Some clients may be able to tell you at the initial interview what they are seeking to achieve, while others may have a hard time verbalizing why they are there and only over time will you begin to understand why they have become clients. But all clients want a therapist to take on the role of being the one with the "power" to meet their needs through the therapeutic relationship.

The therapeutic relationship takes time to develop, and over time clients will begin to trust you if you are sincere and focused on attending to their needs. Because of the power differential, you have the responsibility to shape and maintain the therapeutic relationship. Clients take on a passive role in most cases while receiving massage. For example, a client feels pain in one shoulder, and as you begin to assess the situation, you may ask questions about how the client uses that arm and shoulder. The client feels comfortable telling you that the shoulder was injured while playing soccer with some friends. If you say that the client may be getting too old to play soccer, the client may assume that with your knowledge about the body, you are giving him or her expert advice. The words a therapist uses are important, and we must be careful not to abuse our power as a therapist by judging a client's lifestyle. This client came for pain relief from a shoulder that hurts, not to be criticized for his or her actions leading to the injury.

HOW THE POWER DIFFERENTIAL AFFECTS THERAPISTS

The power differential also affects therapists in a variety of ways. First, it is a large responsibility to develop and maintain the therapeutic relationship in addition to knowing what techniques to use and how to treat the client. Having to pay close attention to all the small details of the therapeutic relationship is difficult for most new therapists, but it is an important component of being a successful therapist. These details may include following up with a client the day after a tough session, following up with a client whom you have referred to another health care provider, gathering information that a client has asked for, or checking into other types of therapies that may help a client.

Second, it can be difficult for a therapist to figure out what the client needs, particularly if the client does not initially give the therapist much information. It can be difficult to read between the lines of what the client says, and this often leads to incorrect impressions. A simple but successful solution to this problem is to check in with your client as frequently as possible. Obtaining feedback from your client throughout a session helps you know how your techniques are working and encourages the client to take part in the healing process. The power differential also gives you the responsibility to care for and maintain the therapeutic relationship, which means that you should seek information from the client and use that information in a responsible way to help meet the client's needs.

It can also be difficult not to take personally what happens with your client. It is not unusual for a therapist to continue to think about something a client said and later feel responsible for some aspect of the client's condition. Most therapists cannot simply end a session and abruptly stop thinking about what the client revealed during the session.

For example, if a female client tells you something personal about her bad marriage and how stressful it is, is it your responsibility to help her fix the bad marriage? Your professional boundaries should limit the extent to which you can help a client, and in a case like this you are limited to helping resolve the client's physical manifestations of the stress caused by the bad marriage. Yet because of the power differential, clients may make you feel like you should provide advice or options related to their personal lives. A better alternative is to help the client through massage therapy to feel better and to offer suggestions such as exercise or meditation to help deal with the stress. It is important to maintain a proper perspective in such cases and know that your job is to work with clients to help them feel better. By helping clients physically, you are also helping them mentally and emotionally.

FINDING THE SAFE AND PROFESSIONAL GROUND

Massage therapists are responsible for learning their clients' needs and trying to meet them. Maintaining a constant connection with the client and obtaining feedback are very important components of the therapeutic relationship. **Assumptions about what we think our client needs, in contrast, can be one of the most dangerous aspects of the power differential with clients.** Every client comes with a need to receive massage, and this need is unique for every client. Some clients may need to achieve a better range of motion, others are recovering from an injury, while still others simply find the relaxation of massage the most positive benefit. A therapist needs to address the client's needs session by session. For example, if a client has been working on increased range of motion during the previous four sessions and comes in after a really stressful week, it may be more advantageous for the client to receive a gentle relaxation massage instead of really vigorous work in this session. Seeking feedback from your clients can help you address what they feel is needed. Most clients come to a session with a goal for how they would like to feel like after the session. Simply asking clients about their goal for the session helps you to begin to understand it.

Ethically speaking, it is not acceptable for you to decide what your clients need. If you have suggestions for a client, an open dialogue is important before the session begins, to help you and the client reach a mutual agreement about the goal for the session. Clients will appreciate you asking and realize you are focusing on them during the session.

Jessie has been receiving massage once a month at a spa over the last 2 years. She has had a number of therapists, and she generally feels most of them have given her good massages. This month, Jessie booked an appointment with a new therapist at the spa. She was told the therapist had been doing bodywork for 12 years, and she felt confident that this would be a good session. When she arrived, she met the new therapist, who escorted her to the treatment room. She was used to talking with the therapist for a few minutes about the goals for the session. But this time the therapist seem distracted and simply told Jessie to get on the table and she would return in a few minutes. After a really tough week, Jessie planned to ask for a simple relaxation massage, but the therapist started the session without talking to Jessie and performed a deep tissue massage. The therapist commented that Jessie's back was really tense and said she would work it out. Jessie felt too intimidated to say anything during the session.

The session ended with Jessie feeling like she had been beat up; she did not feel relaxed at all. Other therapists at the spa had always addressed her needs in their sessions, but this time Jessie was disappointed that her session did not meet her expectations.

On her way out she told the receptionist that she did not want to book any further appointments with this therapist. The spa's manager followed up and asked her for a written evaluation of her session. Jessie felt less intimidated filling out the form than she had talking with the therapist during the session.

In Jessie's case, the therapist did not pay attention to the client's needs but rather had her own agenda for what she felt the client needed. This is a case of a therapist abusing the responsibility implicit in the power differential with a client. The therapist thought she knew what was best for the client. The problem could easily have been avoided if she had talked to the client and listened to the client's goals and needs for the session, then following through with the appropriate work. Ethical principles include making decisions with your clients that will benefit them in a positive way.

As you become more skilled in bodywork, you will more readily understand how to determine what clients need. It will become easier to communicate with your clients and reach a mutual understanding about the goals and techniques for a session. Clients will look to you as the professional to provide information about skills and techniques to be used during the session. Working together with your clients helps them become more involved in the therapeutic relationship and lessens the risk that the power differential may become a problem.

The most effective way to find the safe and professional ground is to communicate well with your client. Verbal feedback from the client is imperative for a good therapeutic relationship. Asking clients about their needs and goals before the sessions starts, checking in with clients during the session, and asking them how they feel near the end of the session will help you address their needs. Clients may also give nonverbal signs of a problem, such as fidgeting on the table, being restless, clenching their fists, or bouncing a foot on the table, when they feel distressed or unhappy with the session. Many clients are not comfortable telling the therapist they are uncomfortable with techniques being performed, because of the power differential. When a client begins to reveal any type of discomfort, it is important for the therapist to check in with the client. Simple questions such as "How are we doing?" or "How do you feel" can open communication lines for clients to tell you what they are feeling. If a client still seems uncomfortable talking about how he or she feels, simply easing up on the techniques you are performing may help the client feel better.

Clients often have trouble communicating with massage therapists during the initial sessions, but showing continual interest in and focusing on the client's needs help form a successful therapeutic relationship. During the interview process it is important to gather information that will help effectively treat the client. It is easy to assume that you understand the information the client has written on an intake form. Asking open-ended questions helps you obtain valuable information that the client may not have written on the intake form. For example, you might make a statement such as this: "You indicated on your intake form that you have headaches. Are these migraines?" A better open-ended question would be, "Can you tell me about your headaches?" The difference in how you ask the question is that the client is encouraged to give you more information than just a simple yes or no answer. Many intake forms are fairly generic, and therapists should take the time to clarify any information needed to effectively treat clients. Likewise, during the session itself, ask open-ended questions to give the client the opportunity to give you more information. For example, instead of saying, "Do you want deeper pressure?" say, "How is the pressure?" and give the client the opportunity to give more meaningful information than just a yes or no answer. Clients do appreciate your interest in meeting their needs.

A client named Rosita was referred to a therapist for injury recovery work after a fall at work. She had suffered lower back injury, and the chronic pain was making it hard for her to stand for any period of time at work. She loved her job and was anxious for her back to feel better.

After the initial intake, the therapist performed some deep work on her back and hips. That evening and next day after the session, Rosita was in intense pain. She called the therapist and asked what she should do. He stated this was a normal reaction and said that she should feel better in a few days. She returned later that week for another session and asked the therapist to work a little lighter so that she would not be so sore. The therapist again performed deep work, and that evening the client could barely move. She called the therapist the next morning to tell him about the pain and was told again that she was having a normal reaction and she would just have to deal with it after each session. She then decided to find another therapist who would be more willing to work within her pain tolerance.

In the case of Rosita, the therapist used the power differential in an inappropriate and unethical manner. The therapist felt that he used techniques that were better for the client over the long term and did not pay attention to or address the client's concerns. The client felt powerless to change the direction of the sessions and therefore ended the therapeutic relationship. This unfortunately can easily happen when a therapist abuses or does not pay attention to the power differential.

Key Points

- Clients look to professionals as experts in what they do.
- Responsible therapists use the power differential in a responsible and ethical manner—serving the needs of clients.
- Communication is an important tool for maintaining a therapeutic balance with the power differential.

DEFENSE MECHANISMS

As mentioned previously, a client or therapist may unconsciously exhibit defensive behaviors during a bodywork session. Clients or therapists may not realize how they are reacting to the work being done or something that the other person has said or done. A client may fidget on the table or move slightly away from the therapist's hands. A therapist may unconsciously begin to feel frustrated with a client. **Defense mechanisms** are involuntary behaviors that unconsciously protect a person or help minimize unwanted or unacceptable feelings and thoughts. When an act, word, or emotion leads to discomfort, we may unconsciously protect ourselves in a variety of ways.

Denial and resistance are two common defense mechanisms for dealing with unwanted feelings. A client may act out toward the therapist, or a therapist may act out toward a client, with neither consciously aware of this. For example, during the session a client might tell a therapist about a friend who is overweight and comment that it is hard to believe that the friend cannot lose weight. The therapist, who has also been trying to lose weight, may react by thinking that the client is in no position to talk because she herself is a little chubby. In this case the therapist displaced his feelings back onto the client, not realizing that he unconsciously felt the client was talking directly to him.

It is important to be aware of the constant interchange of feelings, thoughts, emotions, and energy between you and a client. This interchange begins with the first conversation you have with a new client on the telephone and continues throughout each session. At times you may feel uncomfortable or not at ease with a client, and you might naturally feel that the client has done something wrong. In such a case it is important to examine your feelings and look a little deeper to discover whether it is your own reaction that has led to these feelings.

The interchange between a client and therapist is both physical and psychological. An example of a physical interchange is the work a therapist performs along with the client's reaction to areas that are painful or have reduced range of motion. The therapist may feel spasms or adhesions and then physically adjust the technique being used. The client may feel more pain in a certain area and react by pulling away or saying something. An example of a psychological interchange occurs when the therapist thinks about why the client has a problem or becomes frustrated with a client who is not following suggestions for improving his or her condition. The client may not understand why the therapist cannot significantly improve his or her condition in just one session.

Remember that tissues have memory and store emotion. Some people call these "tissue issues." For example, a client has had a very bad shoulder for the last 2 years, and even with continual therapy the shoulder never feels 100% functional and pain-free for any length of time. The therapist may suspect that some emotional issue is associated with the shoulder, but emotional issues are beyond the scope of practice of massage therapists. It may be appropriate to refer the client to a psychotherapist, but approaching the client about this matter is often difficult. Bodywork can bring a great deal of emotion to the surface, and if a client raises emotional issues during a session, the door may be open for you to make a referral to another health professional. Clients may respond to treatment by crying, seeming sad, giggling, or showing anger, or a client may physically act out and fidget or grab the table. If such a reaction begins, it is important for a therapist to communicate with the client (Box 6-1).

Any time the client shows an emotional and physical reaction, it is important to work only within the client's comfort level. Check in with the client about pressure, pain, and comfort levels. If an area is too emotionally charged or painful, the client will generally tell you that it hurts or does not feel good to have work done in that area.

Clients may also deny that they are having a physical or emotional reaction during a bodywork session. Denying that the work is causing a reaction is a signal that the client is not prepared to deal with the situation. In such cases the therapist should respect that the client is not ready to deal with an issue. Trying to force a client to confront an issue is dangerous and beyond the scope of practice of massage therapy. For example, a client may have a history of some type of abuse, and when certain areas are touched, the client can react emotionally to the physical touch.

A client can become aware that something is causing a reaction. The client may then deny the situation, or may begin to address the issue. Resolving or understanding this can be an ongoing process that may take several days, weeks, or months. If this process hampers the therapeutic relationship, it may be best to refer the client to another health care provider such as a psychologist or psychotherapist to assist the client with emotional issues. Bodywork can still continue through this time as long as the client feels okay with this arrangement.

Remember that a client's reactions to emotional issues are often unconscious, and give the client time to work through the issue. This is an important component of a therapeutic relationship. Forcing clients to cope with their feelings can be very detrimental to the clients. Often clients will feel uncomfortable and not know why, and may not return for future sessions.

Not all tissue memories are related to bad or negative thoughts or feelings of the client. Many memories are very positive. For example, many people just like having their back rubbed because they remember a family member like their mother or grandmother rubbing their back to put them to sleep. There will be many times when clients will relate these to a therapist during a session.

The therapist's defense mechanisms too can cause a client to feel concern or cause misunderstandings. For example, a therapist may be uncomfortable working on a person of another race or ethnic group but may be unaware of his or her own feelings. In such a case the therapist may act out by not focusing on the client or by acting nervously during the session. The client could perceive the therapist's discomfort and may even ask if there is a problem. Typically the therapist would deny that anything is wrong, and both the client and therapist would end the session feeling uneasy.

It is important for a therapist to know that defense reactions such as these are just that—reactions. Yet the client will often notice that something is wrong and will not feel comfortable with the relationship, even though the nature of the problem is unclear. This is a frequent cause for clients not returning for future sessions. Therefore, individuals who practice any type of massage therapy need to be in touch with their own feelings and emotions and thereby prevent defense mechanisms from occurring. This will lead to more successful therapeutic relationships.

> ### Key Points
> - Defense mechanisms are involuntary acts that help minimize unwanted or unacceptable feelings or thoughts.
> - Bodywork can easily trigger defense mechanisms.
> - Communication with clients and feedback from clients can help both parties cope with defense mechanisms.

TRANSFERENCE

Transference is a client's projection of thoughts and feelings about another person onto the therapist. This is a common occurrence and may happen

---

BOX 6-1	*Tips for Checking in With Your Client*

When a client appears upset or uncomfortable, you may ask one or several of the following questions:

- Is that area really sore?
- What is your pain level right now?
- Have you had a recent injury to this area?
- Are you feeling pain anywhere else?
- Would you like me to work lighter?
- Would you like me to stop working in this area?

with your clients in many ways. Transference can occur in any relationship in which you are involved and is generally an unconscious process. Psychologists have suggested that transference behavior grows out of relationships we had in our early lives. Relationships with parents, teachers, siblings, and others close to us in the early years of our lives set the stage for how we react in relationships throughout the rest of our lives. For example, if you greatly respected your father, who was very strong and set all the rules in your household, you may many years later look to a male boss as a father figure who should always be in charge and should be respected in this position. On the other hand, if you had a bad relationship with your father, you may later on react negatively to anyone with that type of influence over your life. In either case, you would have transferred your feelings and thoughts for one person to another.

The very nature of the therapeutic relationship allows transference to happen easily. Bodywork can trigger a variety of emotions from clients such as anger, frustration, sadness, fear, or joy. These feelings are generally the result of some emotion the client felt in the past toward another person. Often these emotions are always present just below the surface of our awareness. Massage can trigger some of these emotions to come to the surface, but also the interaction between a therapist and client can also bring these emotions to the surface. Recognizing that a client's reaction may be the result of transference may help you understand why a client acts a particular way. This understanding can help you maintain a healthy professional relationship. Therapeutic relationships can become unhealthy and negative for either the client or therapist if the therapist cannot cope with this type of situation.

SCENARIO

Angie recently learned about a new massage therapist in her area named Jim, and several friends recommended him to her for massage for her sore shoulder. A college student, she worked part-time on a computer in a small office, and her shoulder ached sometimes when she was tired.

She made an appointment and felt quite comfortable with Jim from the first session. He was about 50 years old and reminded her of her father in a number of ways. This led Angie to believe that Jim could be trusted. After her first session, she felt pretty good. Jim talked to her about some stretches she could do. Jim felt she needed to book at least 8 to 10 more sessions, 1 week apart, to slowly work out all her problems with her shoulder. She could not afford to pay for that many sessions in such a short period, but she really respected and trusted Jim's expertise in this area. She made an appointment for the following

week, but ended up canceling later in the week. Angie trusted Jim but felt confused by the whole situation.

1. Why might Angie have made the appointment instead of just saying she couldn't afford it or saying she would call back later?
2. Were there other options Angie might have explored?
3. Might Jim have been using his father figure "authority" to take advantage of her?
4. What other approach could Jim have taken?
5. Think of a scenario in which both Angie and Jim could have had a healthy therapeutic relationship.

TRANSFERENCE BY CLIENTS

Transference can bring about a positive or negative response from a client. For example, you may respond positively to a person who reminds you of another person who brought you joy or happiness. If during a bodywork session you rub the scalp of a client in a way that reminds the client of his or her mother's touch, the client may feel joy and contentment. Sometimes a client realizes that this is happening and may say something like, "That reminds me of how my mother use to put me to sleep." In most cases, however, the transference is a subconscious feeling or reaction to your touch or something that you say in the session. The client usually exhibits signs that let you know some type of transference is occurring (Box 6-2).

BOX 6-2	*Signs of Transference*

- The client's voice may change (soft, loud, shaky).
- The client's attitude may change.
- The client may begin to laugh or cry.
- The client may tense up or pull away.
- The client may sigh and relax and begin to breathe more quickly or tense up.

Areas of the body that you are working on, the pressure that you are using, or the sound of your voice may remind clients of something from their past. For example, if you talk in a soothing tone that reminds the client of the way his or her grandmother use to talk when she was rocking the client to sleep as a child, this may evoke very positive transference patterns in the client. The client would then likely find it easy to relax on the table during the session. On the other hand, if your voice reminded the client of a teacher that he or she disliked, the client may have a much harder time relaxing while listening to your voice. The tone of your voice during a bodywork session can also trigger a response in the same way. For example, if you talk very abruptly to your client, you may trigger a memory of someone who talked this way to the client at a younger age. If the other person was hurtful, the client may react by drawing inward and not responding well to the session.

Clients generally do not tell a therapist when they are having a negative response during a bodywork session or may not themselves be aware of it. However, they may begin to show signs of retreating, acting uncomfortable, or becoming very quiet. This is why it is important for therapists to check in frequently during the session to learn how the client is feeling. Feedback is essential. Clients are more likely to tell a therapist when a positive transference occurs. If your soothing voice reminds them of a positive time, they may say something like, "Your voice is so comforting—it brings back memories of my dad reading to me at bedtime."

The therapist's thoughts and attitudes can also evoke a response from a client. If you reveal your thoughts and attitudes about a subject about which the client is sensitive, the client may show signs that he or she is uncomfortable. Most of the time, this happens on an unconscious level. Many clients will be aware that they feel uneasy but may not know why. This can lead to the client afterwards feeling the session did not go well or not wanting to continue to work with you.

Knowing that many different situations and scenarios will happen with your clients, you need to be aware of the responses that your clients may have at any time during bodywork sessions. Focusing on your clients' reactions and communicating with them to ensure their comfort will let clients know that you are concerned about their well-being. The therapeutic relationship, therefore, is often the most important aspect of a massage session. The techniques you use and your focus on the client intermingle to help shape the therapeutic relationship.

Receiving positive transference from a client can be very flattering to a therapist. It feels good to receive

---

EXERCISE 6-2

Answer the following questions as if you were a client receiving bodywork sessions from a therapist: How would you feel if the therapist:

1. Talked to you with a harsh tone?

2. Talked in a soothing and soft voice?

3. Talked about a political position that is opposite from what you believe?

4. Made some biased remarks about another culture?

5. Rubbed your abdomen?

6. Massaged your scalp?

7. Rubbed your neck really hard?

8. Hummed during your massage?

After answering these questions, review your answers and consider whether the reason you answered as you did evokes any memories of something or someone in your past. Share some of your answers with your classmates. It can be revealing to see how these different situations can lead to different responses from others.

---

praise and compliments from your clients. Nonetheless, it is still important to manage this aspect of the therapeutic relationship, and this can be challenging for even the most experienced bodyworkers. For example, if you have a client who constantly tells you how good he or she feels after each session and how you are a wonderful therapist, might you unconsciously give better treatment to this client than to your other clients? A situation like this could also become problematic if the client begins to have unrealistic expectations of the therapist. The client might expect to get an appointment at the last minute or on your day off, extra session time, might ask advice on other issues that are beyond your scope of practice, or might step over boundaries by trying to build a more personal relationship.

MANAGING TRANSFERENCE

Transference by the client may occur naturally in the therapeutic relationship in a positive or negative way, and managing both reactions can enhance the therapeutic relationship. Understanding that the transference is taking place and that the client's reactions are related to another person or event can help you avoid taking the reaction personally. For example, if you are working on the upper back and the client suddenly tenses up and becomes very agitated, this reaction may not be from your work at this time but may be a reaction to some past event such as being abused by another person who hit his or her upper back. Words and touch can evoke a dramatic response from a client, and in most cases the therapist has no previous warning that such a response will occur. Most clients do not even realize what is happening when transference occurs. They may feel that the therapist did something or may even deny that they are reacting at all.

Managing these reactions can be challenging for a therapist. The situation should be handled with care. Box 6-3 lists some suggestions when a client begins to show signs that transference is happening.

BOX 6-3 | *Managing Transference*

WATCH FOR:

1. Changes in the client's body (tensing up, fidgeting on the table, making a fist, turning the head from side to side).
2. Changes in the client's emotional state (crying, laughing, suddenly starting to talk or quitting talking).
3. A client asking for special considerations such as changing your schedule or fees.
4. A client trying to socialize the therapeutic relationship, wanting a more personal relationship with you.
5. A client crossing a physical boundary such as touching you too much or needing a hug at the end of a session.
6. A client becoming too personal—telling you too much information.

WHAT TO DO:

1. Check in with the client. Ask how he or she is doing.
2. If the client is physically pulling away, ask the client if you should lighten the pressure or work in another area.
3. If the client is exhibiting an emotional response, ask if the client needs a moment to relax. Sometimes changing the work you are doing will give the client time to process what is happening.
4. If the client is having a serious response, you may ask if the client would like the session to stop and continue another day.
5. If you suspect the issue is overwhelming for the client, a referral to a counselor or psychological therapist may be appropriate. Having a network of referral sources for your clients can help in situations like these. Place brochures or other information in a public place to make it accessible for all of your clients.
6. Keep the relationship professional. When a client starts to cross professional lines, such as asking for your home phone number or wanting an appointment outside your regular schedule, explain to the client what your schedule is and say you can be reached at your office number.

7. If a client becomes too physical, you can avoid being touched. For example, after the session is over, wait behind a desk so that the client does not have the opportunity to hug you. Or, during the session itself, if a client crosses a physical boundary, place the client's hand back into the position needed to continue the session. Usually this physical movement quietly lets the client know you are focusing on the session. If it continues, simply ask the client to stop.

WHAT *NOT* TO DO:

1. Do not try to help the client resolve an emotional issue. This is beyond the scope of practice for massage therapists.
2. Do not tell the client to forget about the issue for now. It may be important to allow the client to work through a response brought to the surface by bodywork. Be supportive but not nosy.
3. Don't be abrupt in your response. It many cases, clients do not realize this is happening. Subtle changes in your approach and demeanor can let a client know that your boundaries have been crossed. If a client does not get the subtle approach, then a direct approach may be needed.

In most of the relationships you form with clients, some type of transference will take place. It is important to realize that this is happening and maintain a proper perspective about the manifestations of transference. Keeping the therapeutic relationship healthy for both the client and therapist is the goal.

Key Points

■ Transference takes place in most therapeutic relationships.
■ Do not take a client's transference reactions personally.
■ Focus on your client's reactions and work in a place that feels both safe for the client and you.
■ Communicate with and obtain feedback from your client.

COUNTERTRANSFERENCE

Countertransference is similar to transference, except that transference occurs from the therapist to the client. Countertransference leads to reactions of the therapist to something the client says or does. For example, if as a child you spent time with an aunt who constantly complained about her boss and you hated listening to her, you may react with the same attitude toward a client who complains about her boss during massage sessions.

The same factors that can trigger a client's transference reaction can also be triggers for a therapist. A client's voice, tone, and attitude all influence how we react to the client. It is important to be aware when this is happening. Box 6-4 lists some very simple signs that suggest countertransference is the reason we may be reacting to a client in either a positive or negative way.

Although the signs in Box 6-4 may seem extreme, countertransference can happen very easily to massage therapists. For example, if you realize that you want to do more for one client than for others, it would be important to examine your reasons for this. If a particular client reminds you of your father and you are going out of your way to receive the client's approval, the dynamics of the therapeutic relationship have changed. Your focus would no longer be on the client, as you become more focused on what makes you feel better. Recognizing that countertransference is happening is an important first step and is something you should consider whenever you feel that something is not right in the therapeutic relationship. The personality of the therapeutic relationship can change a great deal because of this dynamic. The client may begin to feel the sessions have taken on some new dimension and may feel uneasy. Pinpointing the reason for a problematic therapeutic relationship can be difficult unless the therapist is aware of what transference and countertransference look and feel like.

Countertransference can have either positive or negative influence. An example of the positive side is a client who reminds you of someone you care about. In this case your sessions may be more nurturing as long as you stay objective and focused on the client, assuring that the sessions are what the client needs. But if the warning signs listed in Box 6-4 occur, you need to stop and ask yourself if the therapeutic relationship has changed and whether the focus on the client is being interrupted by your own thoughts and needs in the sessions. This does not mean that all positive instances of countertransference result in a negative outcome. Being aware of your reactions and keeping them in check can prevent a negative result. The client may feel he or she is receiving your close attention, and this would feel good. Yet you may actually be paying attention not to the client but to an image of another person in your mind. In this situation your focus on the client has been diverted. What then happens when you become aware of the countertransference and move back in the other direction? Will the client then begin to feel neglected? That is why it is important to pay close attention to your thoughts and feelings about your clients and realize in the very early stages that countertransference could be happening. Knowing that we all often project feelings onto others should help you stop and think before your therapeutic relationship with clients is affected.

Even more than positive countertransference, negative countertransference can be very damaging to the therapeutic relationship. This is a common reason for losing clients. Clients come to receive bodywork sessions to feel better, and if a therapist reacts to a client in a negative manner, the client will likely feel that his or her needs are not being met and may not return for future sessions. For example, a client may remind you of a former friend with whom you are still angry because of some past conflict. Unconsciously, your feelings for this former friend affect your attitude toward the client you are now treating. Your feelings will influence the movement and pressure of your hands on the client. The change may be very subtle. The client may become aware of something negative or may just feel that the session is not what he or she had expected. Although no one can be the perfect therapist for every client who comes into the office, it is important to understand what could be happening in a case like this. Potentially every client you see could remind you of someone from your past. Many psychologists say that all relationships involve transference of some kind. Yet the public expects professional treatment and should not have to be concerned about issues such as boundaries and countertransference. New clients generally do not question what issues you may have unless they have had a bad experience in the past.

Knowing that all relationships can involve transference or countertransference helps you know when something in the therapeutic relationship is not right. Step back and look at why the relationship is no longer focusing on the client, and try to see what behaviors may have triggered your response to the client (Box 6-5). If you do not feel

When the therapeutic relationship is not working, take the following steps:

1. Take inventory of your relationship with a client. List the reasons this person is your client.
2. Write down any emotional issues you are having with the client. For example, "This client makes me angry when he whines about his pain."
3. Think about whether you have had similar emotional issues with someone in your past life. For example, "Aunt Sally always complained about her pain."
4. Try to separate out your feelings or emotions so that the treatment plan is attainable. Aunt Sally may have made you mad, but your client is truly in pain.
5. Remember why the client has come to you. Write down some positive affirmations to use when you work with the client in the next session.

Samuel realized that this was not a good attitude to have with a client and decided to talk to his mentor about what to do. After he explained the case, the mentor asked him if Samuel had dealt with anyone like her in the past, such as a family member. Samuel described how his mother had become very ill and lay in bed for months in pain during his teenage years. His mother not been able to spend much time with him, and he had always resented that she had been sick. Then Samuel realized that he was having similar feelings of resentment toward this client. Knowing that this client had nothing to do with his mother, however, Samuel gained a different way of looking at his client.

In the next session Samuel approached the client with a new attitude. When a feeling of resentment began to creep back in, he easily put it aside, knowing that this client had nothing to do with his past.

you can handle the situation, talk with a mentor or appropriate health care provider about what steps to take to improve the therapeutic relationship.

We never want to lose a client, but it could happen if a client feels something is not right during the session. Talking with the client may be another option, but be sure first that you have figured out why you respond to a client in a certain way. Using the client's time to work out your own problems is not a good option.

Both transference and countertransference can be managed when the therapist is aware of what is happening. As therapists we need to understand when and why it happens. Anytime we lose the focus on our clients, we should consider whether these dynamics may be the reason. Often a simple realization of what is happening can redirect the therapeutic relationship back in the proper direction. If you feel that you cannot manage it, talk with a mentor or health care provider. A healthy therapeutic relationship is rewarding to both the therapist and client.

CASE STUDY

A new client had been referred to Samuel for injury recovery work related to a fall a year ago. The client explained to Samuel that she had a great deal of back and leg pain, and bed rest was the only thing that seems to relieve it. She described her back pain as constantly aching with periods of pain down her legs. While Samuel worked on her, she sometimes cried out, saying that the area was really painful, and fidgeted on the table. Samuel began to find his patience wearing thin when working with this client. She constantly complained about both her pain and other aspects of her life. Many of his suggestions to help her improve were met with opposition, and he felt she could improve much more quickly if she followed his advice. Samuel began dreading his sessions with this client, realizing he always felt physically and emotionally drained after each session. He also found that he had stopped communicating with her and was just doing basic bodywork, thinking that the client just did not want to improve.

Key Points

- A therapist may transfer negative or positive feelings to a client.
- Negative or positive feelings are unconsciously projected to the client through the therapist's hands.
- The therapist should do a self-inventory when the therapeutic relationship is not working or is at risk.

DUAL RELATIONSHIPS

A **dual relationship** occurs when two people have two different kinds of relationships overlapping. Typically, two people have both a social and a professional relationship. At some time during their careers most professionals will experience dual relationships with other business people, clients, or patients. For example, a doctor may meet someone at a social function and form a social relationship. That person may then realize this doctor is appropriate for the treatment of a particular condition he or she has, and then becomes a patient. The doctor and patient thus now have both a social and professional relationship.

Such social relationships are common with professionals and often are very casual. For example, a professional may simply see a client or patient occasionally at social functions. Other social relationships may become more personal, however, potentially causing conflicts between the two relationships. At such times it is good to have guidelines in place for handling situations that can arise, in order to maintain a professional relationship with the client.

CASE STUDY

For the last year, Tom, a massage therapist, had been attending a support group for survivors of cancer. He had met a number of people with whom he related well and had much in common.

One of the members of the group recently injured her back, and her health care provider recommended massage therapy for a couple of months. She remembered Tom from the support group and called for an appointment. Tom asked her to fill out the intake forms as usual. After two sessions he reviewed these forms and realized that she seemed not to have given him full information regarding her back injury. He asked her to provide additional information on the form, but she said that certain information could hurt her case with the insurance company. She asked him to cooperate and withhold some information, adding that the support group members should stick together.

Tom told her that he was ethically and legally obligated to give the insurance company the correct information. She did not return for any future sessions, and later on he found out that she told other support group members he was not a good therapist.

In a case such as this, it is important to inform a client of your responsibilities as a therapist. Withholding information or giving incorrect information to an insurance company is insurance fraud. Your license could be put in jeopardy or a complaint could be made to a therapists' association.

PROFESSIONAL DUAL RELATIONSHIPS

In many types of business, professionals find it is important to network with other professionals in related fields. As you begin to build your own massage practice, you will see that many professionals rely on other professionals in different businesses

to help build their own. Most professionals join business groups to network and gain exposure with others who may need their services in the future. One professional forms a business relationship with another, and each may choose to use the services of the other. Frequently a dual relationship begins to develop as two professionals form a professional relationship after having first met socially and establishing a social relationship. With dual relationships it is important to have clear boundaries. Without boundaries, there is a greater potential for problems to occur that may eventually disrupt the relationship. For example, another professional with whom you also have a social relationship may ask you for a favor or expect a discounted fee from you as a "professional courtesy."

It is always necessary to maintain your boundaries in a business situation. Often this is not problematic. The other person is generally aware that he or she is both your client and a professional associate, and often both of you realize problems can result if boundary issues become cloudy. If the boundaries are not clear, both relationships may end and the other professional would no longer be either your client or your business associate. For example, if you have a friend who is a physical therapist and you have been having problems with your arm, you may ask the friend to take a look at it. That friend, the physical therapist, may request that you see your doctor first. Although such requests may seem innocent, some people do try to take advantage of dual relationships. To prevent problems, professionals generally have to maintain clear boundaries that apply to everyone. This makes it simple and others will see what your boundaries are. This in turn helps you as a therapist avoid decisions that can cause problems later.

CASE STUDY

Gina, a massage therapist building a new practice, joined the chamber of commerce in her town and really enjoyed the regular meetings. She got to know other local business owners and hoped they would recommend her to their customers and associates. She also used local business services as much as possible for printing brochures, maintaining her work space, providing supplies, and so on.

At a monthly chamber meeting she met Veronica, a local bank vice president who seemed to have considerable influence in town. At the next couple of meetings Veronica again talked with Gina, and they seemed to have formed a good friendship. Veronica called her to schedule an appointment. Her back had been bothering her, she said, and she needed some work.

Gina was very aware that a dual relationship had now developed and that she needed to keep the session focused on the client. Yet while Veronica was on the table, she clearly wanted to keep chatting about the chamber meetings and what was going on with other businesses in town. Gina was having a hard time keeping her focus on her work on Veronica's back. She felt pressured to remain friendly and chat with Veronica, but she also wanted to do a good job and thereby keep her as a client and a referral source. Gina knew that if she did a good job, Veronica would feel better and most likely would tell others about her services.

After awhile, Gina told Veronica that she needed her to focus on the massage work they were doing, explaining that she needed feedback regarding her levels of pain and stiffness. She said she enjoyed chatting with Veronica but that now she wanted to make sure they addressed her back problem.

When the session ended, Gina checked in with Veronica to see how she felt. She kept her focus on her client, maintained their professional relationship, did not drift back into their social relationship, which could easily have overshadowed the work. Veronica left feeling her back condition had been addressed and was not upset by the change in focus during the session.

All of your clients, including other professionals, will understand and appreciate it when you stay focused on providing the services they request. Remaining conscious of your clients' priorities will help keep you focused. If you find yourself experiencing a conflict of interest and are unable to keep your focus on the session, as in the case of Gina, you may need to clarify the dual relationship. Communicating with the other party then becomes an important issue before the relationship becomes problematic. For example, if you spend time during sessions talking about the client's business problems, you will not be focused on the bodywork, and eventually this will affect your work and how the client feels about it. Unclear dual relationships can impair your professional judgment and also increase the risk that one party may unintentionally take advantage of the other. The basic guidelines in Box 6-6 can help you avoid situations that become uncomfortable for either party.

Always remember that in dual relationships, each party is seeking something. You may be seeking networking opportunities or using another business for services you need. The other person may also be seeking networking or may need your massage therapy services. This is a give and take situation. Quite often professional dual relationships serve a very good purpose for both parties. Yet, because

BOX 6-6 _Guidelines for Successful Professional Dual Relationships_

- Identify the nature of both relationships (business, social, personal).
- Identify why you have each of the relationships (e.g., a business relationship for networking, and a social relationship since you both belong to the same social group and enjoy each other's company).
- Determine the importance of both relationships to both you and the other professional.
- Identify any potential risks or problems that may arise in the future.
- Work with the client to determine what the focus of your sessions should be.
- Determine ways that you can remain objective and exercise good judgment.

sometimes the dual relationship does not work, you should always be alert for the warning signs of a troublesome dual relationship (Box 6-7). If the dual relationship becomes burdensome and cannot be resolved, it may be time to gracefully back away and learn from the experience.

If you feel a dual relationship is becoming problematic, develop a plan to work it out with the other party before the situation gets out of hand. Effective communication is needed to maintain a healthy dual relationship that remains objective, to clarify the relationship, and to meet the needs of both parties. If the other party is not open to communication about problems you have identified, one or both of the dual relationships may have to be discontinued. A common problem, for example, is feeling that the other person is taking advantage of you. This usually leads to resentment that threatens the professional and social relationship. As always, prevention is better than cure: as you enter a relationship that may become dual, establish boundaries to prevent problems from developing. If they do, try to address them from the start before they become insurmountable.

BOX 6-7 _Warning Signs of a Troublesome Dual Relationship_

A dual relationship may not be working if any or all of the following signs are present:

- The relationship seems one-sided to you.
- You feel you have lost your objectivity.
- A conflict of interest has developed.
- You question whether you are providing competent care.
- You feel vulnerable.
- You have begun to resent the other party.

PERSONAL DUAL RELATIONSHIPS

Dual relationships that involve a more personal relationship are generally more complicated than business relationships because of their very nature as a personal matter. People generally invest much emotion in their personal relationships. Yet it is still important that you set your boundaries clearly for the professional side of the relationship. More often than not, this is a problem for new therapists. As you begin your practice, you may rely on friends and family to help get you started. These people with whom you have personal relationships may become clients and may also offer to help you market your practice by talking with others. This is a great way to get your practice going, but unhealthy dual relationships may develop that could lead to hard feelings with family and friends. Family and friends in some cases will test your boundaries on dual relationships. Be firm but fair, treating everyone the same to avoid problems.

The same basic principles hold true for business relationships and personal relationships. Knowing that there is a risk for conflicts, set your boundaries initially to help prevent problems. Family members may have unrealistic expectations of you and your practice. It is a common problem of massage therapists for friends and family to expect favors. People often assume that because your hands are always with you, they are ready to give massages at all times. Hairdressers often experience the same expectation and are frequently asked to "just do a little trim" while visiting family members. Box 6-8 lists other areas where friends and family members may ask you to cross your professional boundaries.

It is important to address all the boundary issues listed in Box 6-8 with family members and friends. Communicate your boundaries to these individuals and explain that these are important issues not only for you but for the profession. Let them see it is not a personal issue but a professional one.

Discounts for family, friends, and colleagues is a special issue. Many therapists do in fact give such discounts. To prevent problems, should you decide to give discounts, one approach that seems to work well is to give everyone the same discount, such as 20% or 30% off for family members and friends. With a consistent approach no one becomes angry on learning someone else got a better discount.

CASE STUDY

James had moved out of his hometown to attend massage school. After graduation he began working in his new city doing on-site chair massage. Many months later he was looking forward to returning home to see everyone at a family reunion. James put in a very busy work week so he could have an extra day off for a 3-day weekend for the trip home. He had to drive most of the night to make it to the reunion.

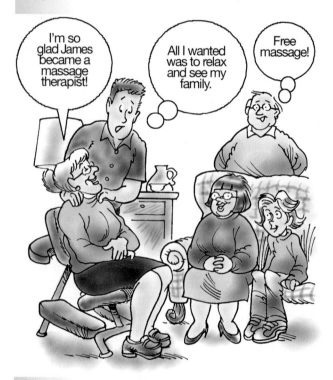

That afternoon, shortly after arriving at the party, an aunt told him she was having problems with her shoulder and neck and asked if he could help her. She said she was miserable but wanted to enjoy the party. James got his massage chair out of the car and worked on her for about 20 minutes. He was anxious to join the party again and see his many relatives, but just as he finished with his aunt, a cousin asked if he could work on her for a few minutes. He could not think of a way to say no, so he started work on her. As others noticed them, a line formed of others also wanting a chair massage. Everyone said they had a special need, and James felt bad for them and could not say no.

BOX 6-8	*Boundary Issues With Friends and Family Members*

- Asking you to give them extra time
- Asking you for a discount
- Asking you to work on days or at times when you normally do not work
- Asking for techniques in which you are not trained
- Asking you to change their records
- Asking you for a massage at their house or other settings
- Asking advice on other health issues outside your scope of practice

Over the next 4 hours James did nothing besides work on family members. When the party ended, he was physically exhausted and had not been able to spend any time socializing with family members except briefly while some of them were in his massage chair. Feeling tired and somewhat cheated out of the reunion, he expressed his disappointment to his mother. She had good advice for him: "Just say no." She advised him to separate his business and personal lives so that people could not take advantage of him.

Most therapists will make exceptions for friends and family members sometime during their career, and often problems do not occur. But if any of the warning signs listed in Box 6-7 become evident, the dual relationship is at risk for failure. This does not necessarily mean that you have to terminate your relationship with the other. Talk with the other party and explain the problem and some possible solutions. If talking about the problem does not resolve it, the relationship may have to be terminated. Terminating a business relationship is difficult, and terminating a personal relationship involves many ramifications on a different level. It may be better to try to maintain your personal relationship and suggest the person see another therapist. Reaching an equitable solution when dealing with family and friends can be difficult unless both parties understand that business and personal relationships are two different entities.

Another dilemma may arise when bodyworkers work with a spouse or significant other. It can be challenging for many therapists to set boundaries with someone who is so close. Students of massage often ask about what to do when they encounter problems. Students frequently report boundary issues with friends, relatives, and significant others. For example, a new therapist wants to show her boyfriend what she has learned at school. The boyfriend wants to talk about personal issues during the massage, and she has difficulty focusing on the session. Often students report that their partners do not understand the true nature of bodywork and try instead to use it as a platform for intimacy, as in the case of Ginny.

CASE STUDY

Ginny came to massage class one day very upset. She told the class that her boyfriend, Andy, was having a real problem with her becoming a massage therapist. Andy felt threatened by the fact that Ginny would be working on other men and wanted her to work only on women. But Ginny wanted to work with athletes and felt such a restriction would be very limiting for her career.

Ginny's teacher asked her what experiences Andy had with massage. It turned out that Ginny was the only one who had ever given him a massage. The teacher asked her how the massage sessions had gone, and Ginny giggled. She said that Andy really felt good and usually ended up wanting to be intimate with her. Ginny admitted she found this fun and sometimes encouraged it.

The teacher then explained that Andy most likely developed his opinion of massage from their own sessions. He probably assumed that Ginny touched all men in the same way. Now that he had formed this attitude, Ginny knew she would have a hard time convincing Andy that things were different with other men.

MAKING DUAL RELATIONSHIPS WORK

Many dual relationships can last a long time and can be very helpful to you and your business, as long as you are aware of them as such and are careful to make them work. Many professionals work within the parameters of dual relationships every day and do not give it a second thought. For example, you may work in the same place as some of your classmates and socialize with them on the weekend. This is a dual relationship. Some dual relationships are very casual, while others involve a great deal of complexity. Competing for clients and tips, scheduling types of treatments, and discounts can all become issues if not handled with care. The same basic guidelines apply in almost all situations to prevent problems from occurring (Box 6-9).

Once you understand that any relationship can develop into a dual relationship, you can see the importance of setting clear boundaries and beginning the dual relationship with those boundaries in place. It is not usually a good idea to make new boundaries, or change existing ones, as you go along. For example, you might give a $25 discount to your first family member who requests a massage. Later you realize you cannot make a living if you give out too many big discounts, so you give the next family member only a $15 discount.

BOX 6-9	*Tips for Maintaining Dual Relationships*

- Know that dual relationships can and will happen.
- Set your boundaries clearly.
- Keep consistent in your policies and actions.
- Communicate your boundaries.
- Be alert for the warning signs of problems.
- Find solutions as soon as problems occur.
- Don't wait and hope a problem will resolve itself.

EXERCISE 6-3

1. Make a list of potential dual relationships that may occur as you begin your business (e.g., relatives, friends, co-workers).

2. List boundary issues that you may need to address (e.g., money, time).

3. List some ways that you can prevent potential problems in dual relationships.

When the second finds out she is getting a lower discount than the first, she is naturally upset. Now do you decide to give them both the $25 discount, along with any other family members who ask in the future, or use a standard $15 discount that may anger the first who had a higher discount? You can see how such an issue can develop gradually or suddenly snowball out of control. To prevent potential problems, start your business with a consistent plan. If warning signs occur, do not wait before looking for a solution. Address the problem as quickly as possible. If you are unsure what to do, talk with a mentor for help finding a solution that is workable for all parties.

Key Points

- Dual relationships will occur.
- Successful dual relationships require boundaries.
- Family and friends may inadvertently test your boundaries and policies in regards to dual relationships.

SUMMARY

Each time you face one of the relationship problems described in this chapter, you will learn a new way to approach similar situations ethically in the future. Some problems can be avoided simply by knowing that the potential exists and setting boundaries to prevent the problems and conflicts from occurring. If a problem does occur, communication is usually your most important tool. Clients look to professionals to be knowledgeable and ethical in all areas involving the power differential, transference and countertransference, and dual relationships. Clients expect to receive bodywork and feel better. It is your responsibility as the therapist to work on all other aspects of the relationship and keep your clients safe in the therapeutic process.

ADDITIONAL ACTIVITIES

1. Pair up with one of your classmates. One is the therapist who is giving a massage to the other, a client. During the massage, the instructor writes different emotions or feelings on the board. No one should speak. For each emotion, the therapist should think about that word and emotion while performing the massage. Experiment with three or four different feelings. After the massage, ask the student who was the client to talk about what he or she felt during the massage. Was there a difference in the massage at various times? How did that make the student feel?

2. While performing a massage on a classmate, try using different tones of voice. Try talking to the client in a soothing manner, a matter-of-fact manner, and possibly even an angry or frustrated way. After the massage, ask the student who was the client how he or she felt at different times during the massage.

SEXUALITY

KEY TERMS

Sensuality: a feeling of pleasure gained from the stimulation of one or more of the senses

Sexuality: the emotional, physical, cultural, or spiritual actions or reactions related to sexual arousal

The massage and bodywork profession was in the past associated in some people's minds with undesirable or illegal sexual activities. The general public is now more educated about massage and bodywork, but as a new therapist you are likely to eventually encounter a few people who believe you are involved in something illicit or illegal, such as prostitution or other sexual acts. Learning how to help others to understand what your profession is and stands for is an important part of your education.

It is also important to understand the dynamics of touch. Touch has many meanings. Your intention as expressed in your touch is an important component in all the bodywork you do. The essence of a massage changes when your thoughts or intentions change. In this chapter, you will explore how your thoughts can affect others.

THE ISSUE OF SEX

The mere mention of the word "sex" evokes many different thoughts and emotions in different people. Our society has strong attitudes about sex, and how and when you were raised influence your own thoughts about sex. It is important to discuss sex and **sexuality** when studying ethics in bodywork because sex is closely linked to touch. Having clear boundaries is an important component of a massage practice.

HISTORICAL PERSPECTIVE

As recent as two decades ago, when someone mentioned the word "massage," others generally associated the word with an illicit act. There were legitimate practitioners of massage, of course, generally called masseuses or masseurs, who often worked in resorts or bathhouses. It was not unusual to get a "rub-down" at the gym, for example. Most of these practitioners worked only with clients of the same gender. At the same time, however, advertisements for massage directed at males, showing female masseuses, were very suggestive—and most people generally assumed that sexual activity was included. Sex for pay was and is illegal in most places, and even when not, referring to prostitution as massage in advertising seemed less obvious.

Legitimate massage therapists who started their practices years ago had to overcome many obstacles caused by this attitude of the general public and law enforcement. Even applying for a business license involved hurdles because local authorities often assumed massage therapists actually wanted to open a house of ill repute. Early practitioners pioneered the way for therapists today, but local and state officials are now more educated about the nature and legitimacy of massage therapy.

CASE STUDY

A group of therapists in Missouri were drafting legislation regarding licensing for massage therapists. When they felt they had a viable proposal, they hired a lobbyist to represent them in the state legislature. The lobbyist did his homework and found that a state senator had recently proposed restrictive legislation about massage. It seems that in his town a number of businesses provided massage, but unfortunately these businesses were fronts for a sexual trade. His proposed legislation would give each county the right to ban any type of massage from being performed in that county, as he wanted his own county to do. This senator truly believed that the word "massage" meant sex.

The group of therapists and lobbyists asked for a meeting with the senator to discuss his bill. After a 2-hour meeting, the senator had a completely different view about the practice of massage therapy. He learned about the education required for becoming a therapist and the important role of bodyworkers in the health care system. The therapists agreed in turn with the senator that businesses should not be allowed to use the word massage to cover for sexual trade. Together they vowed to pursue legislation to allow legitimate massage therapists to work and to require anyone using the words "massage" or "bodywork" to be professionally trained and certified. That legislation passed and now stands as a law good for the public and massage therapists alike.

Movements to pass legislation and educate the public about massage have dramatically changed the public's view of massage. Advertising in newspapers, magazines, television, and radio describes the benefits of massage. To attract the public to their facilities, resorts and day spas advertise massage as one of their key features. Mention the word "massage" now, and most people will think of how they could really use one to relax or feel better. Associations such as the American Massage Therapy Association (AMTA) receive more than 5,000 calls per month from the public and therapists requesting information about massage. The AMTA media center has become a well-known source for information about massage. This group and others like it help educate the public not only on the benefits of massage but also on topics such as the qualifications of therapists, differences among massage modalities, and current legislation and ethical issues. Both experienced therapists and new massage students will continue to change the public image about massage and bodywork.

Every bodyworker has the responsibility to act professionally and ethically at all times. Practicing in health care carries a great deal of responsibility. Being a bodyworker is not simply a job—it is who you are. For example, when you see your doctor in a social setting, you still relate to him or her as your doctor. In many professions individuals have a professional persona they carry everywhere. Doctors, accountants, nurses, managers, and business owners all relate professionally to others in many settings. Massage therapists fall in the same category. This is why it is important for all therapists to understand past attitudes toward massage and know that with each bit of education we give others, we are furthering the profession for ourselves and others who follow.

Although the past poor reputation of massage has generally faded, sexuality still remains an issue in the massage community today. Touch can evoke sexual feelings and thoughts in both the client and the therapist, and therapists need to be aware how this can happen and how to handle such situations professionally and ethically.

PROFESSIONAL BOUNDARIES AND SEX

Because of past attitudes toward massage, professional therapists see the need to maintain clear boundaries regarding sex. In the past, legitimate therapists wanted to distinguish themselves from others who performed illegal acts under the name of massage, which resulted in associations writing codes of ethics and states including wording in laws and regulations addressing the sexual issues. Boundaries help therapists know where the line is between professional and unprofessional behavior, and boundaries have also helped the public understand what massage therapy really is. The codes of ethics discussed in Chapter 3 all set boundaries regarding sex. Most ethics codes state that therapists will have no sexual contact with clients. Many states have rules and regulations further defining what specific contact is or is not allowed. For example, a law may state that no massage can be performed that involves touching the genitals of a client. This is a fairly clear rule to follow.

State laws, rules, and regulations also define the process by which a client may allege that sexual touch occurred and the consequences of such allegations. For example, the rule may state that a person can file a complaint in writing. The complaint will be heard and investigated by the state board, and if the therapist is found in violation of a rule, the board may suspend the therapist's license to practice. State and local ordinances similarly define the parameters in which a therapist can practice. Some of these definitions involve ethical issues to help therapists and the public know the boundaries.

Boundaries can involve sensitive issues, but many professions have boundaries related to ethical issues. Mortgage brokers, for example, have associations and state laws that address ethical issues. Because of past infractions involving clients' money, these issues are controlled through codes and rules. Boundaries remain a public issue in the bodywork profession because some individuals still try to hide behind the words massage or bodywork to perform illegal acts. This happens more frequently where laws or ordinances are lacking or are not enforced.

Acting responsibly, educating the public, and feeling comfortable as you work in your profession all help others who may still be skeptical understand that massage is a valuable and integral therapy for maintaining health and well-being.

Key Points

- The public image of massage and bodywork has significantly changed over the last two decades.
- Legislation and education have been key factors helping the public understand the massage profession.
- Every therapist should be part of the process of continuing to educate the public.
- Boundaries help to clarify sensitive issues.

THE DYNAMICS OF TOUCH

Touching another person always involves an intention of some type and evokes a response. You may express happiness or sorrow by hugging someone, or playfulness by tickling or wrestling, or nurturing by rubbing someone's shoulders. The other person knows the meaning you are transmitting not only by the type of touch but also by your intention expressed in the touch. When you are happy and hug someone, for example, the hug is generally uplifting, but when you are sad the hug may be more clinging and involve other motions such as rubbing. Generally the other person can feel your intention and responds to that intention along with the touch itself. Sometimes, however, the other person may not understand your intention and may react in a way that shows he or she is not in sync with you. When this happens, the other person may have difficulty handling what you are offering or may reject feelings of any kind at that moment.

Massage is generally considered to be a nurturing type of touch. People make appointments for massage in order to feel better or reduce stress and to take care of themselves. Therapists convey to clients through touch and words what their intentions are. Unfortunately, some individuals may confuse the nurturing with other thoughts or actions that could be sexual in nature.

THE MEANING OF TOUCH

How a person responds to touch involves the individual factors discussed in Chapter 2, Values and Emotions. People react to touch and intention according to their own values and beliefs, which are mostly formulated during their early years. Someone who was brought up in a home where touch was a part of everyday life may naturally feel very comfortable receiving a massage. An individual who was raised in an environment where touch was not prevalent, or where touch may even have been associated with punishment, may not feel comfortable receiving a massage. Remember that not everyone thinks of massage in a positive way. Some people may object to having someone else touch their body, especially in situations such as occur with massage. Clients who are new to massage can be unsure and hesitant about the experience. It is important for therapists to recognize this reaction and treat clients with respect. Every person has a comfort zone, and clients should never be forced to go beyond their comfort zone. Undressing and having another person touch their body can be very uncomfortable for some. They may understand that a massage would feel good but cannot get beyond their emotions about getting undressed. Such clients may be good candidates for a chair massage, allowing them to receive positive touch under conditions they feel more comfortable with. Others may not feel comfortable at all having another person touch them in any way, perhaps because of past experiences of abuse or punishment or because of their own perspective of their body.

Remember too that body tissues can hold memories of pain, emotions, or trauma. A therapist should never force a client to go beyond what the client feels comfortable with. It is important to respect clients' thoughts and feelings during a massage.

Therapists encounter a wide variety of reactions to touch from clients during bodywork sessions. Some clients may perceive the therapist's touch as sexual even though the therapist does not have any such intention or feelings. A client may, for example, find being touched on the abdomen or thigh a trigger for sexual feelings. Therapists can be surprised by a client's sexual reaction and need to be prepared if it happens. This does not mean that a therapist has to constantly be aware of touching all parts of the body in fear that a client will react. Rather, therapists should be aware of any shift in the client's behavior, and if it becomes evident that the client is reacting negatively or sexually, the therapist should change the work, pressure, or area to avoid embarrassing the client. The client's reaction may surprise the client as much as it does the therapist. Changing the routine can help eliminate the reaction in many cases. If an inappropriate response continues, the massage session may need to be stopped.

It is also important to recognize differences in how men and women sometimes relate to their feelings and to touch. Men tend to associate touch and sexuality more commonly than females. Some men have issues with other males touching them and may request a female therapist. A new therapist may feel uncomfortable when a male client specifically requests a female therapist. Touch is a personal experience for the client, however, and the client should feel comfortable with the gender of the therapist. Some therapists too may feel more comfortable working on one gender because of their own safety zone. It is important for therapists to explore their own feelings about clients of both genders and their own preferences.

EXERCISE 7-1

Think back to your first days in massage school and try to recall if you felt some hesitation with any gender issues. Respectfully discuss with your classmates how you and they felt then, and try to understand how your clients may feel the same way. Discuss ways that you can address these issues with clients.

CASE STUDY

Veronica had received three massages from John over the last couple of months and had really begun to enjoy the effects of the massage. At her next appointment, she mentioned to John that she had a stiff neck and shoulders and would like to concentrate the work in that area this session. As he worked, she began to feel her upper body let go and begin to relax. When John began work on the front of her neck and shoulders, using deeper pressure right under her jaw line, she felt her shoulders tense up. John also noticed it and asked Veronica to take some relaxing breaths. He again worked along the jaw line and noticed that Veronica was much more relaxed and even had a slight smile on her face. She seemed to cooperate much more this time and even commented that touching that part of her neck felt really good. John assumed that he had just touched a sensitive spot and that she reacted to that sensitivity. He continued to work in the area. Veronica began to breathe a little heavier and even moaned a little when he worked up by her ear. John then realized that Veronica's reaction to his touch had become more sexual than therapeutic and knew he needed to change the course of the massage. Not wanting to embarrass her, he moved back down to the shoulder, changed his pressure, and worked on trigger points in her shoulders. Slowly Veronica returned to the focus of the session and likely did not realize that John had noticed her earlier reaction.

As the dynamics of touch are wide and diverse, it is important to always be aware of the client's emotions and reactions to touch. The therapist's intention may be to eliminate tension in a certain area of the body, but the client could respond to touch in a more sexual way. Therapists cannot know in advance what may trigger a client's reaction, but it is important to take notice of a client's change in demeanor or attitude. Changing the routine, pressure, or area generally eliminates an inappropriate reaction. If an inappropriate response continues, the session may need to end.

Sometimes a male client may react to touch by developing an erection. The first time it happens, most therapists are usually very uncomfortable and unsure how to handle the situation. The client may be embarrassed by the reaction and not understand why it occurred. Some may not even realize that it has occurred. Changing the focus of the routine to incorporate a different pace, area, or pressure can help. In some cases it may be appropriate to explain to the client that touch can lead to many different reactions and that working in some areas can evoke responses. It also may be appropriate to say nothing at all, particularly with a client who seems unaware of this response.

DIFFERENCES BETWEEN SEXUALITY AND SENSUALITY

The words sexuality and sensuality are often linked in our society. **Sensuality** is a feeling of pleasure gained from stimulation of one or more of the senses. People find different things sensual, and they also vary in how strongly they respond to sensual stimuli. Sensuality is only partially under conscious control—we can choose to have a sensual experience, but we cannot "choose" to feel pleasure from it. That is a result of a person's past experiences and is part of what makes us human and an individual. For example, smelling the aroma of a food that you really love can be a sensual experience. Movie scenes of a beautiful waterfall can evoke sensual feelings. Touch can also be a sensual experience because touch is one of the senses. An aromatherapy massage given in a warm room with soothing music involves three of the senses, and many find this a sensual experience.

Sexuality can be similar to sensuality in that it involves pleasurable feelings that may be directly or indirectly related to the senses, but it is different in that sexual experiences generally evoke sexual arousal whereas sensual ones do not. An experience may be both sensual and sexual at the same time, such as a certain kind of caress, but the sensual dimension itself although pleasurable doesn't cause arousal—that comes from the sexual dimension. Exercise 7-2 can help you understand differences between sexuality and sensuality.

EXERCISE 7-2

For each action, write down whether you think it could evoke a sensual or sexual response.

1. Touching a baby's face

2. Looking at a beautiful painting

3. Holding hands with a significant other

4. Receiving a note thanking you for your kindness

5. Kissing your significant other

6. Massaging a good friend

7. Smelling your favorite dish cooking

8. Massaging a client's back

9. Hugging your best friend

All the actions in Exercise 7-2 generally evoke some type of response. Understanding such responses relates to therapists' responsibilities during bodywork. Some clients find all touch sensual. Touch often evokes a response that is sometimes emotional for some people, sometimes sexual for others.

COMMUNICATION THROUGH TOUCH

When students are asked at the beginning of their bodywork training why they want to work in this field, most say it is because they want to help others. That is truly a good beginning. What most students do not realize at first is how much attention needs to be paid to the multiple dimensions of massage to become a good therapist. An important component is the communication between the therapist and a client.

Throughout a massage session several types of communication occur. Verbal communication occurs when you interview your clients, talk with them about different massage modalities and techniques, and check in with them about their comfort level during sessions. Therapists may also explain massage modalities or boundary issues they feel are important.

People respond to touch much as they do to words: they may understand exactly what the therapist intends or they may react differently because to them the words or touch carry some other meaning. Touch is a form of nonverbal communication, involving what some call "gut feelings" or intuition. Nonverbal communication occurs both from therapist to client and client to therapist. If your intention during a massage is to provide a totally relaxing session, your hands will convey that to your client with long, soothing strokes that nurture the client's well-being. Most clients find this very relaxing, but a client could respond to this massage sexually. Attentiveness to the client's nonverbal communication is just as important as the techniques you are performing (Fig. 7-1). Being proactive and focused on the client help you stay tuned to the client's nonverbal communication, which can help you prevent uncomfortable situations from happening. For example, if you feel a client is reacting inappropriately to a certain technique or area you are working on, you can change to another technique or area to change the client's reaction.

The therapist's intention is also important. What is your intention when you hug your best friend? You are not trying to evoke a sexual response but are simply sharing your feelings with a friend, such as showing that you care. But even

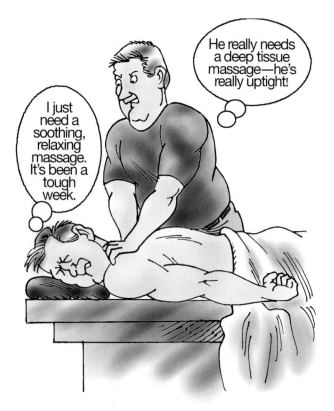

FIGURE 7-1 ■ Paying attention to the client's nonverbal communication will help you know how the client is reacting and when changes are needed in your technique.

when you do not intend to evoke a sexual response, another individual might respond in that way. Both intention and response are involved in a complex dynamic in bodywork. The therapist and the client both come to a session with a goal in mind. The therapist should ask the client what his or her goal is for the session, and this helps the therapist set his or her own intention for a session. The client then responds to that intention and the work being done. The intention and responses are present before, during, and after the session. Constant verbal and physical communication helps the session be successful. Therapists who do not stay in "sync" with a client, whose intentions do not evoke the appropriate responses, often find that the client leaves the session feeling that the massage was not very successful.

Ethically, a therapist has stepped into a danger zone when his or her intentions become tainted. If a therapist steps outside professional boundaries and begins to think in an inappropriate way about a client, the client can feel that intention. For example, if you begin to think about how attractive a client is, your hands and thoughts will have a changed intention. Your hands may begin to move in a more seductive way, perhaps even without you realizing what is happening. Negative emotions and thoughts can also affect intentions.

For example, if you are frustrated by a client who is always a few minutes late, those feelings can be transferred to your hands and the client may feel something different during the massage. The client may feel that you are rushing or being a bit rough with your strokes. The intention of your touch can be influenced by even the most subconscious thoughts and feelings.

An integral part of training in massage is to learn to be in touch with your own thoughts and feelings and to understand that at times you will need to refocus your intentions. Problems and feelings from the world outside can affect your touch and therefore what a client feels in the massage. Train yourself, before each massage, to take the time to focus on your intention for that massage. It can be challenging to stay focused throughout the session, but whenever you realize that you have lost your focus, make the effort to bring yourself back to the session and focus on your therapeutic intention for it.

CASE STUDY

Jamie had already performed six sessions today and was feeling quite tired. She had a busy evening planned with her family. A few minutes after the scheduled time, her last client still hadn't arrived, and she felt her frustration rise because she knew she had to leave the office right at 5:30. Her client finally showed up, late due to traffic, and while doing the massage, Jamie found herself thinking about having to hurry to the store because she was running late. She would fix a quick dinner because she had to be at a school play by 7:30 for her oldest daughter's first acting performance. She was very excited to see the play. Then she suddenly realized that she was in the middle of a massage and could not remember if she had done both of the client's feet yet. With effort she refocused on her client, feeling bad that she had for a while lost her intention for the massage. At the end of the session, the client remarked that she did not seem herself today. Jamie commented that she had had a long day and must have been tired. Jamie knew her client had felt her loss of focus during the session.

Key Points

- Every form of touch has an intention behind it.
- Clients can unconsciously or consciously feel your intention.
- Intention is just as important as the techniques or routine.

SEXUALITY AND TOUCH

New therapists are often very surprised when a client responds sexually to their touch. For example, working on the inner thighs may evoke sexual arousal in some clients. How do you prevent this? First, refocus on your intention for the session. If you feel the client is still reacting inappropriately, changing the pressure or technique can help. Otherwise, leaving the area is appropriate. Many areas of the body may evoke a sexual response. Therapists cannot always know when this will happen and should therefore be flexible enough to change the routine or move to another area as needed. Most clients would be embarrassed by their response and would prefer it if you did move on with the routine.

Although this is a delicate topic, it is important to consider what happens when a client becomes sexually aroused. A female who becomes sexually aroused may begin to move her torso or hips on the table. She may rock back and forth. A male may respond similarly and may develop an erection. Depending on the client's position, you may or may not see this happening. Both males and females may sigh or moan. If any of these signs appear during a massage, change the area where you are working or take a short break from the routine. It may be enough just to check in to see how the client feels. If necessary, talk with the client to see if he or she is aware what is happening. The client may not be consciously aware of how he or she reacted to the massage, and will likely be embarrassed. If the client is aware of the sexual response and wants to continue, this is the time to explain boundaries. If you feel the session is no longer under control, stop the session.

After such an experience you may feel shaky and unsure if you handled the situation in the most appropriate way. If you experience a situation like this and have difficulty coping with the feelings and thoughts that result, talk with a mentor.

SEXUAL ATTRACTION

Sexual attraction can happen anywhere and at any time—this is simply a part of human nature. A human response such as sexual attraction to another person is natural and can happen even when the focus is on bodywork. It is important, however, to recognize when sexual attraction is appropriate and when it is inappropriate. Many professional ethics codes state what is considered inappropriate. Similarly, many companies have policies that personal relationships between employees in the workplace are not acceptable. Sexual harassment has become a major issue in our society and leads to many lawsuits. Doctors and health care practitioners are especially vulnerable to being accused of inappropriate behavior. If a client pursues a more intimate relationship with you, it is important to remember your professional and sexual boundaries. Do not allow the massage session to become a forum for pursuing any type of relationship other than a therapeutic one. Likewise, if a therapist has feelings outside the boundary of a therapeutic relationship, pursuing these feelings during massage sessions could be considered sexual harassment by the client.

Touch is associated with sexuality and a bodyworker's job is to touch others—in an appropriate way. Again, consider that your intention for a session can and will be felt by the client. If you find a client attractive and begin thinking about that during a massage, the intention of the massage may change from one of relaxation and healing to involve a more sexual touch. Your hands will reveal what your mind is thinking. Because bodyworkers are in close physical contact with clients, it is easy to admire a client's body whose characteristics you find attractive. Professional therapists can understand that the client's body has physical beauty but still maintain their focus on the therapeutic goal of the bodywork and the tasks for the session. Focusing on techniques and outcomes helps maintain the ethical relationship. If you find you cannot control your feelings, however, it would be important to talk to your instructor or a mentor before the situation gets out of hand. When a therapist cannot control his or her feelings, the therapeutic relationship should end. The therapist should explain to the client the issue of professional boundaries and refer the client to another therapist.

During a session, conversation may take place. In most cases such conversation with the client should be limited, allowing the client to relax. A client who does not understand what is going on during a session may talk out of nervousness. If so, you should pay close attention to a client's state of mind and try to reassure the client about the session. For example, a client who has never before received a massage and who feels nervous while you are draping the leg may start talking about something completely out of sync with the massage to avoid thinking about your actions. The client may just be feeling nervous and vulnerable about having the leg exposed. Explain to the client that you will be working the top part of the leg and that the draping will prevent uncomfortable exposure.

Therapists should always be aware of what they are saying during a session. Even a casual remark can be taken in the wrong way and lead a client to incorrect conclusions about your intent or actions. Jokes and comments about sexuality are inappropriate in the therapeutic relationship. Part of your training involves learning to filter your comments carefully so that the client feels comfortable. Even long-time clients can become uncomfortable with a therapist because of an inappropriate comment.

Either the therapist or client may feel sexual attraction in a bodywork session. Recognizing your own feelings or those the client is exhibiting is an important first step for acting responsibly and ethically. Focusing on the intention of the session is the second step. If you cannot control your thoughts or feelings, the ethical and responsible thing to do is refer the client to another therapist.

EXPLORING YOUR OWN SEXUALITY

Talking about sex and sexuality is often uncomfortable for massage students and beginning practitioners. But examining your own thoughts about sexuality helps strengthen your foundation and make any needed changes in order to practice ethically.

Chapter 2 discussed the values and morals with which we were raised and how these have a tremendous influence on how we act and react to clients. In Exercise 7-3 you are now asked to write down your thoughts about certain aspects of your own sexuality. Many of these thoughts are very private, although you may choose to share them with your classmates. You may be surprised to find that others have similar thoughts.

EXERCISE 7-3

Write a sentence or two about how you feel about each of the following actions, situations, and thoughts.

1. Being touched in areas such as the lower back, upper legs, and gluteal region

2. Touching others on the lower back, abdomen, chest, and gluteal area

3. What makes touch sexual?

4. At what point does touch become inappropriate?

5. Can I hide my feelings from a client?

6. How do I feel if a client is attracted to me?

7. Have I ever had inappropriate thoughts about others while performing a massage?

8. What did I do about it?

9. What should I do about it?

Exploring your own thoughts about touch and sexuality can be very helpful for beginning a career in bodywork. Students who do not understand this part of their psyche can end up not being prepared to handle thoughts and feelings they may feel at times as well as clients who may react to touch in a sexual way.

Key Points

- Sensuality and sexuality are often linked with touch.
- Perception of touch is influenced by a person's background, upbringing, and past experiences.
- Recognition of inappropriate thoughts, feelings, words, or touch is an important step for professionals.
- Talk with a mentor to understand your feelings or the reactions of clients.

ISSUES INVOLVING SEXUALITY

Issues involving sexuality that a bodyworker may encounter are those involving a client's action or sexual reaction to bodywork and those involving the therapist's own thoughts and feelings about a client during bodywork.

MANAGING CLIENT ISSUES

A client's reactions during massage may occur very innocently and naturally. The massage therapist's gentle, nurturing touch could be unconsciously misinterpreted by a client. For example, if a client's husband often rubs the back of her neck while expressing affection, she may respond to that touch as being sexual in nature. Most therapists would not think that touching the client's neck could be a trigger for an emotional response, but you should constantly monitor a client's reactions during bodywork sessions to become aware of such responses. Being conscious of the client's responses to your touch is an ongoing process. If you feel a client is reacting in a way that is not appropriate, for example, simply changing the technique, pressure, or area usually stops the reaction. If the reaction continues, it would be appropriate to talk with the client to bring the client back to an awareness of the goals of the session. But if an inappropriate reaction occurs that cannot be managed this way, the session should be ended. A therapist has the right to refuse to treat a client if the therapist determines that the therapeutic relationship cannot be maintained in an ethical manner.

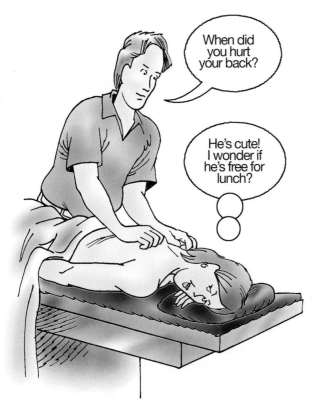

FIGURE 7-2 ■ The effects of a gentle touch may lead a client to feel attracted to a therapist. The therapist needs to be aware of the client's response and adjust the technique accordingly.

A more problematic issue occurs when a client is sexually attracted to a therapist. This may be a natural attraction or the result of transference. The transference of a feeling for another person or the effects of a gentle, nurturing touch could lead a client to feel attracted to a therapist (Fig. 7-2). The client may reveal his or her feelings through subtle or sometimes blatant remarks or movements. Once the therapist is aware of this happening, a change of the routine or techniques may prevent the problem. But if the client continues to show an attraction to the therapist, it is appropriate to talk with the client and suggest a referral to another therapist. Because the therapist and client are alone in a room together in most cases, it is imperative to take precautions to prevent any improprieties from happening. Improprieties include a client making a sexual suggestion or comment, touching the therapist, or making any type of advance.

The most extreme issue is a client who consciously expects bodywork to be a sexual experience. This may happen with a client who has had no experience with massage therapy and who naively believes the old myths that once associated massage with prostitution or illicit sex. Obviously, a massage session with such a client will be problematic and should be ended immediately when the client's expectations become evident. Box 7-1 lists safeguards to help prevent an uncomfortable or potentially dangerous situation from happening.

Usually you can screen out inappropriate clients over the phone. A potential client who asks questions about things like what clothing the therapist wears or makes suggestive comments about feeling especially good after a massage may have a different expectation for the session. Simply tell the client you do not do that type of work and hang up. It is not professional to call the person a name or make other inappropriate remarks.

If a client seeking sexual stimulation does happen to make it into your facility, trust your intuition when you begin to feel something is wrong. If you feel uncomfortable with the client, remember your foundation. If you stay strong, the client will not be able to intimidate you. If a client makes suggestive remarks, tries to remove the draping, or makes sexual movements with his or her body, simply tell the client the session has ended and the client must leave. Taking payment for a session that you end this way is at your own discretion. Some feel that this person has taken their time and should pay for the session, while others feel that would be accepting money for what the client intended to be inappropriate behavior. Therapists should follow their own guidelines with which they feel comfortable. Ideally, other people are present in the office or nearby, making it unlikely that such a client will cause trouble. But if you truly feel threatened, call the police. Avoid seeing a new client late in the evening or when you may be alone in the building. Take steps to keep this from happening, and maintain some control over your schedule. For example, if you work in a salon where a receptionist books your appointments, you can let that person know that you do not work on a new client for your last appointment of the day without prior approval if there is any chance you will be the last one in the salon and might be left alone with the client.

As well, keep in touch with other therapists in your facility. Often they can tell you about a client who has behaved inappropriately, because some clients go from therapist to therapist to see what they can get away with. Note, however, that many laws, rules, and codes state that information about clients must be kept confidential, and sharing this information may be against the rules. To help protect therapists, facilities may maintain a list of clients who are not welcome to return for therapy. If you have had a problem with a client, it would not be ethical to tell others about it; this is unfortunate because this client could try the same thing with other therapists. The problem is becoming rarer as the public becomes better educated about what massage therapists do.

CASE STUDY

Josh had opened his massage practice in a chiropractor's office a couple of months ago and was seeing an average of 15 clients a week. He practiced 3 days a week when the doctor was in the office and had begun to see clients also on Saturday when the doctor was not there. The doctor referred a woman who expressed an interest in massage. Josh made an appointment for 2 o'clock on Saturday afternoon.

After the intake, he showed the new client the massage room and explained his routine. The client was very friendly and commented that she was lucky to have such a handsome therapist. Josh thanked her but thought to himself that this was not appropriate. During the massage, the woman talked a lot, often putting her hand on Josh's arm while she spoke to him. Josh asked her several times just to breathe and enjoy the massage and said that he was having a hard time focusing on the session while talking so much. Eventually the woman asked Josh if he would be interested in having a drink after the session. Josh knew she was crossing the line and told her that he could not socialize with his clients. She again touched his arm and said she had not been touched like this in a long time. Josh told her that comments like that were not appropriate. The women commented that just the two of them were there and no one else would ever know what happened in that room. The session then ended, and Josh was relieved.

Then the women asked to book another session for the following week. Josh declined. He said that she would have to find another therapist. He did not feel comfortable working with her and understood that another session with her could lead to trouble.

BOX 7-2 | *Managing Attraction to a Client*

1. Change your focus. Your client is there to receive bodywork.
2. Think about your ethical obligations. Your clients and your peers expect you to follow ethical codes and guidelines.
3. Talk with a mentor. Talking through your feelings and thoughts with another professional can help you understand what is happening. A mentor can also be more objective about the situation.
4. Refer the client to another therapist. If you cannot work through your feelings, referring the client is the most professional thing to do.

MANAGING THERAPIST ISSUES

An issue that does not get media attention is how to approach your own sexuality when working with another person (Box 7-2). With a significant other, you may already have a history of sexuality that most likely involves touch. In other words, you yourself may sometimes associate touch with sexuality. This can be especially difficult if you have given massage to your significant other that led into sexual activity, making the association still stronger. A related potential problem is that your partner may associate the touching of massage with sexual touching and therefore assume that things might get out of hand when you are giving massage to others. It is important to educate friends, relatives, and significant others about the intention that therapists need to maintain a therapeutic relationship with clients. Others may joke about what happens on a massage table and even have suspicions about inappropriate behavior. Helping others understand the seriousness and focus that is required can take some work, but in the end they should understand what is required of a therapist. Sometimes you may need to invite them to receive bodywork in order to see the professionalism that occurs while a client is on the table.

Box 7-3 offers some suggestions to help others in your life understand your work and the professionalism you need to be successful.

BOX 7-3 | *Maintaining Professionalism*

1. Have a clear understanding with others that this is your work and your profession. Socializing and personal feelings are not part of a session.
2. Think of your table as your office.
3. Concentrate on your work and not on other issues.
4. You can control the session. If you feel you cannot, stop the session.

Inappropriate feelings, thoughts, and behaviors can occur with any client in your practice. Acting on such feelings or thoughts is dangerous and an ethical problem. Some state regulations and codes of ethics include guidelines therapists must follow in this area. Even having inappropriate thoughts during a session is problematic because your hands may naturally communicate such thoughts to your client. It is important always to stay focused on the session and therapeutic relationship.

At present, most states do not have clear-cut laws, rules, and regulations that specifically address the issue of massage therapists dating clients, although some ethical codes do refer to this behavior. It is a difficult situation when an attraction develops between a client and therapist. If you really are attracted to a client, your mentor may suggest talking with the client and referring the person to another therapist.

CASE STUDY

Jana had been practicing massage for 8 years, and her full-time practice was thriving. She saw as many as nine clients a day, and she loved her work. It was rare to find a spot for a new client, but a client had recently moved away, and a regular had referred a man named Mike to her. She instantly liked Mike's sense of humor. After their third session, Mike asked Jana if she had time to go to lunch. She told him she was fully booked that day and did not have time. She knew she could not go out with a client but was just trying to get herself off the hook and let him down easy. She did think, however, that if the circumstances were different, she probably would go out with him.

During the next session, Mike again pursued the issue of going out. This time he asked her to dinner. Jana told Mike that she did not date clients. Mike said nothing for a few minutes and then jokingly told Jana that she was fired—so now he was not her client. She did not know what to do. He told her that although he really liked his massages, he would be willing to find another therapist so they could see what happens.

Jana did not work on Mike anymore. She did begin to talk with him on the phone, but still did not feel comfortable going out with him. After about 6 months, Jana felt she could begin a relationship with Mike, and they then dated for 3 years.

Consider the case of Jana and Mike. Why did Jana feel she had to wait a while before beginning a relationship with Mike? She had two reasons.

| BOX 7-4 | *Best-Kept Secrets* |

If you find any of the following happening to you, talk with a mentor or instructor:

- If you have mixed feelings about a client or begin to question your intentions in the massage session
- If you find yourself thinking about a client in any way other than in terms of massage techniques and the treatment of the client
- If you talk to someone else about a client in any but the most professional way

First, she did not want other people to view her actions as an impropriety. Some people might think, for example, that getting a massage is a good way to get to date a massage therapist, and this attitude would likely encourage inappropriate behavior. Second, Jana wanted to make sure of her own feelings for Mike. She understood that a momentary emotional attraction felt for a client might not be a true basis for a relationship and that it was too easy for her simply to rationalize her feelings. We humans can always easily justify those actions we want to take, if we're not thinking about the ethical consequences.

Sexuality and socialization are part of who we are, and learning to separate our personal and professional lives is important. People in many professions have to face this issue, but bodyworkers are especially vulnerable because touch is an integral part of what we do. Bodyworkers are not alone, however, in facing the challenges of working with others. Psychologists work with the human mind, and doctors and nurses also work with the human body. Many health care professionals frequently face dilemmas with their clients. Personal values and morals, as well as the effects of the power differential in the therapeutic relationship, can make that relationship very complex at times. It is natural and human to have thoughts and feelings about others, but it is professional to know how to act and react when such situations arise.

Key Points

- Touch evokes a large array of issues.
- Be aware of any client reaction.
- Be proactive in handling a situation.
- Talk with a mentor or other professionals if you need guidance.

SUMMARY

The therapeutic relationship involves a wide array of complex variables that may develop. Being aware of potential problems and knowing how to manage issues that may arise help a therapist handle situations that could become inappropriate or unhealthy for either the client or therapist. Talking with a mentor or instructor in the early stages of a potential situation helps prevent problems from developing. Approach every therapeutic relationship with a mind-set focused on what is appropriate, and you will find it easier to create a healthy therapeutic relationship for both you and the client.

ADDITIONAL ACTIVITIES

1. Look up a code of ethics for another profession, including other specialties in health care. Look for any references to dating clients or related inappropriate behaviors.
2. Ask friends and family members if their profession has an ethics code. If so, how has this code affected their behavior? Have they ever experienced a situation with the potential to violate their code of ethics?
3. Of the ethics codes that you have seen thus far, write down two code statements that seem the most important to you to prevent inappropriate behavior involving sexuality.

8

DISCLOSURE

CHAPTER PREVIEW

- Disclosure is sharing information with other health care providers or your clients
- Client disclosure of information about their health history for the safe practice of massage
- Nondisclosure of information placing the client at risk during massage
- Third-party disclosure is a health care provider sharing information with another party
- HIPAA regulations guaranteeing the information rights and responsibilities of patients and health care providers
- Therapist disclosure of information regarding treatment, outcomes, credentials, and personal health issues to clients
- Ethical behavior involving knowing the boundaries related to disclosure

KEY TERMS

Disclosure: revealing information to another person about oneself or another person

Third-party disclosure: giving information about a client to an outside person

The word **disclosure** as used in the health care professions refers to sharing information. Clients disclose personal information to massage therapists about their health, therapists disclose information to clients about the treatments and modalities they use, and therapists may also disclose information about a client to a third party such as an insurance company.

Disclosure involves several ethical issues. Using a client's information only in a safe and ethical manner is an important principle bodyworkers should safeguard and maintain. To practice ethically, it is equally essential to give correct information to clients about their treatment and the modalities to be used in a session. This chapter examines these and other issues related to the disclosure of information and problems that may arise.

CLIENT DISCLOSURE

When potential new clients call to book an appointment for bodywork, they generally do not think about the information they may need to share before receiving a massage. Clients typically are thinking of the benefits they will receive from the bodywork, such as relaxation or pain relief. But the benefits often depend on the massage therapist having certain kinds of information about the client.

NEED FOR CLIENT DISCLOSURE

Bodyworkers ask complete strangers to disclose a great deal of personal information about their health history before receiving treatment. Often new clients are somewhat surprised with the amount of information that a therapist asks for before a session begins. Most therapists have new clients fill out an intake form that asks questions about medications, past surgeries, and any medical problems they have or have had in the past. A client who has received massages before may be familiar with the intake form. New clients, however, may feel uneasy disclosing their personal health information to a bodyworker. Therefore, it is important for a therapist to explain to new clients the need for this information and the safeguards that will be taken with it. A client's health history is used to assess any signs, symptoms, or other information that suggests there may be contraindications for massage or that help reveal what massage techniques may be most effective for the client. For example, with a client taking a pain medication, the therapist should ask if the client took the medication prior to their session. If so, no deep or invasive work should be done because the client cannot give accurate feedback. Explaining this to clients helps them understand that you are looking out for their best interests and that there is a need for this type of information on their health history.

CASE STUDY

Hector had never received a massage before. He was referred by his doctor for bodywork for the low back pain he had experienced over the last few weeks. He made an appointment with Kimberly and was asked to come a few minutes early to fill out the paperwork. Hector was somewhat surprised to discover that he had to fill out several pages of forms and diagrams before the session could begin.

Kimberly noticed his apprehension and sat down with him while he was filling out the paperwork to help with the questions. She explained that information about his health could help her treat him more effectively and, more importantly, prevent any inadvertent harm during the session. She showed Hector a textbook that listed contraindications for massage and bodywork. She told him she took her job very seriously and that she wanted to treat him knowing as much relevant information as possible. Kim also reassured Hector that his health information would be kept confidential and shared with other health care professionals only if he gave her permission to do so. She explained that if he wanted the treatments and progress shared with his referring doctor, she would first ask for his written permission.

Educating clients is an integral part of being a bodyworker. Therapists should not assume that clients will instantly trust us and understand our expectations for them. It is often necessary to carefully explain to clients that in your training you learned that massage could sometimes be dangerous to a client's health or condition. For example, if a client tells you that he or she has been experiencing shooting pains down the leg since a fall, that client should see a medical doctor to be evaluated. Doing bodywork in such a case could make the client's condition worse.

It is important to differentiate between a client's medical history and signs and symptoms stated by a client. The medical history can include a diagnosis that was made by another health care provider. For example, a client may write on the health history section of the form that he or she has high blood pressure and colitis. These conditions most likely were diagnosed by a medical doctor. The same client's signs and symptoms may include achy joints, back pain, fever, and numbness. It is the responsibility of the therapist to ask questions about these symptoms to assess whether massage may be contraindicated. For example, if a client at present has a fever, a massage should not be performed. If a client has back pain, the therapist should seek further information by asking questions: Has any medical condition been diagnosed affecting the back? When did the pain start? Where precisely is the pain? What is the pain level? One client with back pain may say that she saw a doctor and was told it was arthritis, and that her pain level was pretty low except when she did heavy work. Another client with back pain may say he fell yesterday and feels a sharp pain shooting down his legs. You can see the big difference a few questions can make when assessing a client's condition. The client with an arthritic condition could have some work done, whereas the client with a more acute condition after the fall should be referred to a medical doctor for further evaluation.

If a therapist discovers signs, symptoms, or conditions that contraindicate massage, the client should be informed that medical evaluation may be needed. Clients often ask a therapist to diagnose what is wrong with them. Diagnosing is beyond the scope of practice for bodyworkers and massage therapists. It is easier to explain to clients with a diagnosed medical condition why they cannot receive bodywork. It is more challenging to discuss this with clients experiencing signs and symptoms but who do not have a medical diagnosis, because these clients typically want to know what you think the problem may be. Tell the client that there are certain signs and symptoms that may indicate conditions that a massage therapist should not work on. If the client asks what condition you think is present, it is best to say that as a massage therapist you cannot try to diagnose medical conditions and the client should seek medical advice.

The therapeutic relationship must be handled with care, compassion, and professionalism. Talking with clients about the importance of this information may ease their concerns about supplying some information. Every therapist should have at least one reference book in the office to check possible contraindications when needed and to educate clients when questions arise. Show your clients this reference material pertaining to their diagnosed condition if needed to demonstrate that you are concerned with their well-being. Ruth Werner's *A Massage Therapist's Guide to Pathology*, 3rd ed; Lippincott Williams and Wilkins; Baltimore, MD; 2005 for example, is a good reference for therapists to look up conditions with which they may be unfamiliar. It can also help clients understand why their condition is of concern to a massage therapist. Clients who understand how possible harm could result from a massage or certain modalities will appreciate your concern as a professional and trust that their best interests are truly important to you.

How much information clients are asked to provide about their health varies from nothing at all to a multiple-page intensive health history. Some salons and spas use the same intake form for clients receiving haircuts, manicures, facials, and massage. Some of these forms ask no questions about the client's health history. In some practice settings, various other forms can be used, including pain questionnaires, injury reports, and updates of information. As a bodyworker, you need to decide what information is important for you to have in order to treat a client effectively and safely. Questions about medications used, surgeries, and diagnosed conditions should always be asked before any bodywork is done. Additional information regarding symptoms such as level, location, frequency, and duration of pain, numbness, weakness, fever, and areas of redness will help a therapist assess whether clients may have underlying conditions that could result in harm with therapy.

Health history forms are available from many different resources. Fig. 8-1 includes a sample form that can be used in practice. Other sample forms can be found in massage and medical textbooks. Many therapists like to customize their own forms that organize information in a format they find convenient. Others design their own forms to ensure they have all the information they may need in reference to all rules, regulations, and laws affecting their practice.

When designing your own intake form, consider what information you need to treat your clients safely and effectively. High blood pressure, contagious diseases, and inflammatory disorders are all important conditions therapists must know about before treating a client. Put yourself in your clients' place. Would they feel some of the information you are requesting is too personal? Do you really need to know this information? Why? Anticipate that clients may wonder about these things while they are filling out your forms. Some clients may ask why you need certain information, while others may feel some information is not relevant and simply may not disclose it to you. Communicating with and educating your clients can help them understand the importance of the information you are seeking and reassure them that you are striving to provide the safest and most effective treatment. You can include a brief explanation on the intake form itself or talk with clients before they fill out the intake form. Some therapists even mention the importance of this information in their brochures. It is important for clients to trust that you are providing quality treatment and that you will safeguard their information in a confidential and ethical manner.

CLIENT NONDISCLOSURE

Some clients may not disclose certain information for one of the following reasons:

- The client does not feel comfortable sharing the information.
- The client does not think certain information is relevant.
- The client forgets to disclose something specific.

Clients may refuse to disclose something because they feel the information is private. Personal issues may be involved, such as past abuse or disturbing emotional memories associated with a condition. A client may also need time to develop trust in a therapist before disclosing personal information. This information may or may not affect the massage treatment being given. At times this information may not be relevant to the client's physical condition but involves an emotional issue for the client. For example, a client who has been treated for depression may not feel a massage therapist needs to know about that in order to give a massage.

In some situations clients may not list a condition that would put them at risk when receiving bodywork. Massage therapists therefore must learn signs and symptoms that indicate something is wrong. For example, while working on a client's leg, you notice red streaking going up the leg. When you question the client, she tells you her leg has been sore for the last couple of days. The streaking and soreness could be signs of a blood clot or thrombus, which is a serious condition and would contraindicate massage. Explain to the client what you have observed and that she should see a health care professional for a diagnosis and care.

In such cases clients usually ask you what is wrong. Tell the client that you cannot give massage because of the signs and symptoms, although it is beyond your scope of practice to diagnose the condition. If you suspect a client may have a medical condition, you are within your rights to ask the client about his or her health and any diagnosed conditions. Some individuals ignore their symptoms and

Client Intake Form

Name_____ Date_____

Address_____

City, State, Zip_____

Home Phone_____ Work Phone_____

Occupation_____

Referred By_____

Current Health History

Are you currently being treated for any medical conditions? Yes___ No___
If yes, please explain_____
_____

Are you currently taking any medication? Yes___No___
If yes, please list the medications and what they are for.
_____
_____

Please list any surgeries or injuries and the dates when they
occurred_____
_____

Have you received massage before? Yes_____ No____
Please list any areas of complaint that you would like addressed during your
session(s) _____

Please circle any of the following conditions that apply to you. These may be conditions
that you currently have or have had in the past.

Muscle/Skeleton	Digestion	Other
Headaches	GERD	Hearing Loss
Pain in Your:	Indigestion	Visual Loss
Back	Constipation	Diabetes
Neck	Irritable Bowel	Fibromyalgia
Shoulders	Diarrhea	Cancer
Arms	Crohn's Disease	Eating Disorders
Chest	Colitis	Caffeine Use
Abdomen	Gas/Bloating	Nicotine Use
Glutes		Alcohol Use
Legs	Circulation	
Feet	Stroke	Skin
Arthritis	Blood Clots	Rashes
Bursitis	Varicose Veins	Allergies
Scoliosis	Heart Condition	Acne
Osteoarthritis	High Blood Pressure	Warts
Tendonitis	Low Blood Pressure	Psoriasis
Joint Disease	Swelling	Dry/Oily Skin
Sprains/Strains	Lymphedema	
Fractures		Reproductive
	Respiratory	Pregnancy
Nervous System	Asthma	Current
Numbness/Tingling	Sinus Problems	Past
Radiating Pain	Shortness of Breath	PMS
Paralysis	Hay Fever	PID
Chronic Pain	Fainting	Endometriosis
Herpes/Shingles	Pneumonia	Hysterectomy

Please list any other diagnosis that applies to you that is not listed above.
Please indicate if you are still being treated for this condition.
_____

I have disclosed all known conditions and diagnoses that I am aware of and
verify that all the information above is accurate. I understand that a massage
therapist will not diagnose any conditions and will keep the above
information confidential unless receiving a signed release from me. I will
inform the therapist of any changes that may occur in my health history.

Signature_____ Date_____

FIGURE 8-1 ■ Client intake form.

do not understand the need to see a health care professional. If you see an indication of a serious condition, do not alarm the client but suggest that the client call a health care provider soon. For example, if you see a dark mole on a client's back with irregular edges, tell the client what the mole looks like and say that a medical professional should check the mole and see if it is cause for concern. Helping clients understand the importance of recognizing when their health is at risk is a responsibility of all health care providers. Take care, however, not to scare a client or say what you think may be wrong (diagnosis). Educating clients demonstrates that you keep their best interests in the forefront.

CASE STUDY

Today Maryann was seeing a new client, Andi, who had found her in the yellow pages. Andi explained that her back had been hurting for the last couple of weeks and that she wanted some work in that area.

When Andi arrived, she was anxious to get on the table. Maryann asked her to fill out the health history form before they started. Andi said she just wanted some work done and said she'd fill it in later. Maryann explained that she needed the information to effectively treat her in the session today. Andi reluctantly filled out the form, but Maryann had the feeling she had skipped over some sections in her health history.

Maryann decided to do an interview before they began. She asked Andi how long she had felt the pain, if she had experienced anything that might have caused her pain, and what her pain level was. Andi said that she had had a very heavy menstrual period that lasted 10 days. She said her pain was pretty intense, especially the last few days. She said that she had not been able to see her doctor and just wanted the pain to go away. Maryann asked if she was running a fever, and Andi said her temperature had been 101 to 102 the last couple of days.

Maryann then knew she could not work on this client. She needed to educate her, instead, about the importance of seeing a health care provider. Maryann told Andi that because of her symptoms, she should not have a massage until she had seen her health care provider. She explained, for example, why massage therapists should not work on clients with a fever.

Andi became very upset and asked Maryann what could be wrong with her. Maryann explained that she could not try to diagnose her condition. The fever and the pain suggested something might be wrong that required medical attention, but she couldn't even speculate about it. She did know, however, that massage could possibly make her worse. Maryann therefore encouraged Andi to call her doctor right away to ask for an appointment.

Andi called Maryann a few days later. She said that her doctor had discovered she had a uterine infection that now was being treated. She thanked Maryann for recognizing that she should have this condition taken care of, and said she would be back to see her when her condition was cleared.

In the case of Andi, the therapist could have ignored her signs and symptoms and performed the massage anyway. Instead, she acted ethically by referring the client to her doctor to ensure that she received appropriate care.

Clients sometimes glance over the health history form and feel some of the information you are asking for is not relevant, and they therefore may not disclose this information. This attitude results when clients do not understand why this information is important. This situation can be prevented by a brief paragraph on the form telling clients why this

EXERCISE 8-1

With the class divided in three groups, each group discusses one of the examples below. List possible solutions for your example situation. Each group then reports its findings to the class, and everyone discusses any other possible solutions.

Example 1: A new client has filled out a health history form listing no major illnesses or surgeries. In the signs/symptoms section, he writes that he is often tired, has abdominal pain, and lately has often felt nauseated. What do you do?

Example 2: A client has filled out a health history form, and you see nothing written there that would contraindicate receiving massage. The client's only complaint is upper back and shoulder pain. While giving the massage, you see the client has a large scar on his chest. When you ask the client about the scar, he says that he had open heart surgery 4 years ago. Then he asks why you want to know about his surgery and how it is relevant to a massage for minor pain. What do you do?

Example 3: A new client has been referred to you for low back pain caused by a recent fall at work. The client reports that she finds it hard to work because her pain is so severe. The doctor's report states the pain is caused by muscle spasms. During the treatment session, the client reports that she also has had back pain for about 5 years, especially after doing heavy lifting. When you look over the client's intake form, you see that she wrote that her only back pain was recent. When you ask her about this, she says that she forgot about the other times when her back was sore and says she thought the form asked only about her recent pain. What do you do?

information is important or by talking with clients before they fill out the form.

If the client has not completed the form accurately, you may notice subtle clues during the massage that lead you to suspect that the client left out information. For example, many people have experienced some type of whiplash in a car accident. The effects of whiplash can last for many years, and clients may not realize that their neck or shoulder pain may have started with the accident. During the massage they may remember that their pain started not long after the accident. A therapist can then ask questions about medical treatment or any diagnosis made at that time. Therapists need any information that can help treat clients effectively. Knowing about clients' conditions may very well affect the massage techniques used. Help clients understand why this information is important. Clients often comment that they did not think a particular condition was relevant to massage. Explain why the information is important, and update the information on the client's form. Asks clients before every treatment about any changes or updates in their health or conditions.

Finally, some clients may simply forget to disclose information. When one is filling out a form, it is easy to forget an illness or accident, especially something that happened some time ago. Clients may not think to include their broken arm when they were a teenager or their appendix being removed when they were 20. Yet their present signs and symptoms may suggest a condition you need to know about. You are within your rights to question clients further when their signs and symptoms may be relevant to treatment. Educate your clients about the importance of your having this information.

In any case in which a client does not disclose information, massage may involve inherent risks. Clients are usually unaware of the importance of disclosing their health information to a therapist. Box 8-1 lists ways you can help ensure clients disclose important information.

If you make every attempt to obtain all relevant information for the treatment of a client, you have acted in an ethical and professional manner. Clients do have the right not to disclose information, but they should be educated about the risks of receiving bodywork if so.

Key Points

- Disclosure is an important part of bodywork.
- Decide what information you need to treat clients effectively and safely.
- Communicate with and educate your clients about the importance of disclosure.
- Clients may choose not to disclose information.

BOX 8-1 · *Helpful Hints to Ensure Client Disclosure*

1. Include a brief paragraph on your health history form explaining the reasons for asking about clients' health.
2. Look for clues in the client's answers on the health history form, such as fever, fatigue, soreness, etc.
3. When in doubt, ask the client questions during the oral interview.
4. Watch for signs and symptoms that could mean the client has a condition that could contraindicate massage.
5. Keep good notes and records of your session with clients. You may see patterns develop that need further investigation.
6. Ask clients at the beginning of each session for any new information about their health.
7. Include on your form a statement that the client has disclosed all known health information. The client should sign and date this statement. This helps prevent clients from knowingly not disclosing health information, and helps protect you legally if the client has not disclosed a condition that could become worse with massage.
8. Always be honest in recording information that you have learned. Clients have no argument with a professional who is honest.

THIRD-PARTY DISCLOSURE

Third-party disclosure is giving information about clients to another party. Third parties may include medical doctors, osteopaths, chiropractors, insurance companies, physical and occupational therapists, or lawyers. You may also receive information yourself from other parties about your clients. For example, if a chiropractor refers a client to you, you may receive information pertaining to the condition that you are treating.

Medical professionals may refer clients to you and then request information back about the client's progress or current status during treatment. Even when a client is referred to you, you still must have permission from the client to share any information. Other health care providers may also need to know past treatment information about a client, including what modalities were used, assessment information, and outcomes of the treatment.

In all of these cases, **the client must give written permission for you to share the information about the client.** This is most frequently done using a consent form (Fig. 8-2). You have probably signed such a form yourself at a health care provider's office. The information could be for an insurance company or another health care provider. The consent form includes the client's name, with whom the information will be shared, and the client's signature and date. Spoken permission is not acceptable and could be risky for the therapist. A client

---

Client Consent Form

I, _____, give my consent for Therapeutic Associates to release

my treatment and health information to _____.

_____   _____

Client Signature   **Date**

FIGURE 8-2 ■ A typical consent form.

could later say that you did not have permission to share the information and you would have no proof; it would be your word against the client's.

New patient privacy legislation has taken effect in recent years, and as health care providers, massage therapists need to adhere to the same guidelines all other providers follow. The Health Insurance Portability and Accountability Act (HIPAA), which became effective in 2001, protects consumers' rights to privacy of health and health care information, nondiscrimination in health care coverage, and the rights of consumers regarding shared health information. All health care professionals must follow these regulations. Detailed information about HIPAA regulations is available from the U.S. Department of Health and Human Services, Office for Civil Rights, on the Internet at www.hhs.gov/ocr/hipaa. Clients need to trust you with their health information and to know that it will be shared only with their consent. If you share information without a client's permission, you have crossed an ethical boundary and may be denying the client's legal rights.

In addition to HIPAA, your state's laws, rules, and regulations may dictate what information you must keep about each of your clients and how long records must be kept. Some states require little or no record keeping, while others are very specific about what information is required and the confidentiality of clients and their records. Check your state laws and rules to assure that you are keeping all necessary information about your clients and know how it can be shared with other parties. You can customize your office forms to make this easier.

Insurance companies are third parties that may request information about modalities or treatments used for a client, the length of sessions, and outcomes. It is important to know what specific information the client's insurance company may need in order to pay a claim. If necessary, contact the customer service department or claims adjuster to learn what information you need to send, after the client has given you signed permission to do so.

Lawyers may also seek information about clients, such as when a lawsuit has been filed regarding an injury for which a client is being treated. Lawyers may want detailed information about client assessments, session information, outcomes, and costs. If questions arise, check with the lawyer's office, preferably in writing, asking what specific information is needed. If you know a legal case is involved, make this inquiry early in the client's treatment to prevent having to write notes from memory later on. Dates of treatment, specific client complaints, and outcomes are particularly important when litigation is involved. Obtain written permission from the client to share this information. In some cases such information may be subpoenaed.

Insurance companies and other health care providers usually do not request detailed narratives of your sessions with a client. Some want a beginning assessment, a statement of modalities used, and the client's outcome or progress. Some may want only an overview of what happened with the client. If you are unsure about the exact information to provide, ask the third party what specific information is needed. Insurance companies will return or deny a claim if information is missing.

Although third-party disclosure of information seems pretty straightforward and easy to understand, ethical situations or questions can arise in some areas, such as in the scenarios in Exercise 8-2. In such cases it is important for therapists to know their boundaries and the importance of maintaining ethical standards.

Some clients will test the therapeutic relationship from time to time. Clients may ask you not to report something to another health care provider or an insurance company. Other health care providers may ask you to provide treatment but bill under a different procedure code to ensure payment. Situations like these can be perplexing to a new therapist. It is intimidating to have to tell a doctor that you cannot falsify the nature of a client's injury or treatment for billing purposes. When faced with an ethical dilemma, check what rules, regulations, and laws affect you. Consult an attorney, if needed, if

EXERCISE 8-2

With the class divided in three groups, each group discusses one of the examples below. List possible solutions for your example situation. Each group then reports its findings to the class, and everyone discusses other possible solutions.

Example 1: A chiropractor refers a client to you after a car accident. The client is receiving treatments from both of you each week, paid for by his insurance company. Then the client complains of additional pain in an area that had not previously been affected and wants work in that area too. What do you do?

Example 2: A client has been receiving treatment for the last 6 weeks for pain and lack of movement in her right arm. Her insurance company approved a series of eight treatments. At the end of the eight sessions, you feel you have done as much as you can, even though she still has some pain. The client asks you to report to the insurance company that her pain level is still fairly high and she needs six more treatments. What do you do?

Example 3: You have a new client who wants to be treated for a car accident injury. She reports that she is suing the other driver for her injuries and asks you to keep good notes for her attorney. After each session, she wants to read your notes. After the third session, she does not like the wording of some of your notes and asks you to change what you wrote to make her pain sound more extreme. She feels this will help her case. What do you do?

you have a question about insurance fraud or falsification of client records, which are both punishable by law.

The notes that therapists and other health care providers keep about clients have involved some controversy. Some feel that this information belongs to the providers, while others feel clients or patients have the right to all notes about them. What a health care provider writes can be read by others, however, including the patient or client, insurance companies, other health care providers, and attorneys if litigation is involved. Therefore, all information must be true and accurately reported. Even casually written notes can become legal documents, and you should write all client notes keeping that in mind. If you choose to talk to another party about a client situation, such as when seeking assistance from a mentor, be sure not to use the client's real name unless you have written permission to do so; just call the client Jane or John Doe.

> ### Key Points
> - Consent is required to release client information.
> - Check what information the third party needs.
> - Know your legal responsibilities.

THERAPIST DISCLOSURE

As a therapist, you provide clients with information about the modalities and treatments you perform, your credentials, and your own health. Educating your clients about the modalities and expected outcomes helps them be part of the process of reaching their goals. Clients also need to trust your credentials and training and to know that they are not at risk for health problems by interacting with you.

DISCLOSURE OF MODALITIES AND TREATMENTS

Clients who are being treated for a condition or injury frequently ask about certain modalities and what they can do for them. Many also ask how long treatment will last and how quickly they will get better. In most cases, unless a client specifically asks for a certain type of work, the therapist determines what type of bodywork best suits the client's needs. One client may benefit most from deep work such as myofascial release, while another may gain more from craniosacral therapy. Therapists should discuss with the client the work to be performed along with expected outcomes.

Most bodyworkers have learned a variety of massage styles to serve their clients' needs. Schools of massage offer a large and diverse assortment of massage styles. Many students begin with Swedish massage or Shiatsu as a foundation for their education. The time spent learning a specific technique can vary from 2 or 3 hours to hundreds of hours. Because of such variations, students often wonder at what point they can say they are proficient with a particular technique. Is it after a few hours or a few days of instruction, or should it take several months before advertising a specialty technique? This question has long been debated among even the most seasoned massage practitioners. Instructors who are qualified to teach a technique (having received the appropriate education) can usually tell you how many hours of instruction you need before you are proficient enough to advertise performing a specialty technique. Students can also research other sources of training information, such as any pertinent state laws or regulations, and ask other practicing therapists what qualifications or training is needed to perform specialty techniques. You may also need to check any state laws, rules, and regulations about what qualifications may be needed to advertise a technique or modality.

Once you are satisfied that you have reached the appropriate level of education and skill in a technique, have practiced many hours, and feel confident that you understand the technique and know the results, you can tell clients that you are trained in that specialty. Clients may still ask how many hours of training you have or how long you have been using a particular technique, and your answer should be honest.

Massage therapists should continue to attend education seminars, read books, and research specialties. New information is constantly available about the effects of different modalities. Some modalities with different names are very similar treatments but involve slightly different approaches. Research these modalities, and ask other therapists if they have attended courses. Your clients may even tell you about other techniques they have received and the results of those sessions.

When you treat clients with specific techniques, you have the responsibility to tell them what they should expect from the treatment. If the type of work may leave a client sore for a day or two, it is your obligation to inform the client about that before your perform the technique. Clients should always have the choice about what they receive. For example, clients who are told that a certain type of massage may leave them sore for a few days may choose not to have that work done now because the timing is bad for other activities in their life. Before the session begins, explain the modality, what the client should expect during the treatment session, and the expected outcome. Clients have the right to refuse treatment if they feel this type of therapy is not for them. You may offer the client other options, such as other types of massage, or a referral to another therapist who does another type of work.

With all modalities, clients should be taught about appropriate uses for the technique and expected outcomes. If a client asks a question regarding a modality or treatment and you are unsure of the answer, do not be afraid to say that you do not know, but then take the time to research the answer and get back to the client as soon as possible. The client will appreciate your concern. It would be unethical to make up an answer just to give the impression of being knowledgeable or to justify a treatment. Ethical treatment of clients includes providing correct information.

DISCLOSURE OF CREDENTIALS

Clients often ask where you went to massage school, how long you attended classes, and how many hours of education you have. Questions like these are usually fairly easy to answer, since most students' initial education is usually clear-cut. But describing how you have continued your education in new and different modalities can be much more complex.

Bodyworkers attend seminars and conferences to learn new approaches and styles of massage that interest them or that clients have requested. Continuing education courses are offered on single weekends, over several weekends, or over many days depending on the class. Some educational sessions involve a small amount of information or a simple technique. Others contain a great deal of information and complex techniques. At what point can you ethically say that you perform this new technique? In the massage community there is something called the "weekend warrior" syndrome. A therapist may attend a weekend seminar in a specialty technique and on Monday start telling clients that he or she is trained in the new technique. Weekend workshops frequently involve a great deal of information and offer some time for hands-on techniques, but they seldom give enough practice time for one to become proficient in a new technique. Many such courses also do not test the proficiency of participants to ensure they can perform the techniques in a safe and proper way for clients.

Ethically speaking, therapists who attend weekend workshops should take the time to practice their new techniques and research more fully the information presented in the seminar. Would you want a surgeon practicing on you on Monday after just learning a technique in a weekend seminar? Only when you feel confident that you fully understand a technique, are skilled in performing it, know its effects, and can truly educate your clients about what to expect, should you advertise the new technique. Ideally, instructors of these workshops and classes should test their participants before allowing them to advertise the new specialty. Many educators are moving in this direction and have developed courses with different levels of proficiency for students.

You may have seen bodyworkers advertise that they perform as many as 10 different types of massage or bodywork. One may wonder how proficient a therapist may be at so many different types of work. Specialties like craniosacral therapy take a great deal of education, time, and practice to become proficient. A weekend workshop just introduces a small part of what is needed to perform this type of work. Yet some therapists feel justified in advertising each and every workshop they have attended. The ethical issue here is that a client could potentially be misinformed about a therapy or, even worse, hurt by a therapist who is not trained sufficiently. Many people do not know to ask therapists how much training they have before receiving the work. Therapists should become proficient in any technique before advertising or working on clients with the new technique. Work with the instructor or other therapists to improve your skills before working with clients.

Some facilities advertise having many different types of massage available. This is common in spas or salons. Their menus may include deep tissue, sports, aromatherapy, Ayurvedic, reflexology, and hot stone massage. Ethical businesses hire therapists who are trained in these techniques and book clients requesting a specific technique only with an appropriately trained therapist. Unfortunately, some businesses claim that all of their therapists are trained in all techniques and give therapists only a crash course in a technique. Educating business owners is also an important aspect of being an ethical practitioner.

New massage school graduates are sometimes hired into unethical practices such as these, and you should be aware this can happen. The spa business is growing very fast and is highly competitive. Therapists should not perform techniques in which they are not trained; if a client asks you for such a technique, talk with your employer. Before accepting a position, ask your potential employer what techniques you are expected to perform. Many spas will provide in-service training in some of the specialty techniques. Client safety is always essential, and all businesses and therapists must be qualified and trained in the techniques they practice.

DISCLOSURE OF HEALTH STATUS

Therapists expect clients to inform them about their health and any conditions they have, to help determine if massage is safe to perform. Clients should also expect their therapist to disclose any information that could affect them adversely. For example, if a therapist has a viral infection such as a cold or the flu, clients should be informed. Most facilities have or should have policies regarding employees who have contagious conditions, typically stating that appointments are to be rescheduled until the condition has passed. The decision whether to continue practicing generally depends on the level of risk to the client. If a therapist has an infected sore on the arm, for example, it could present a risk during bodywork. Yet the same sore on the leg, covered by a bandage and clothing, may present minimal risk.

Our world is affected by a number of serious long-term communicable diseases. Herpes, Hepatitis B, and HIV are examples of serious contagious viruses. The Centers for Disease Control and Prevention (CDC) has tracked the number of health care workers affected by diseases such as HIV/AIDS since the 1990s. For example, in 2001, 5.1% of the more than 450,000 reported cases of AIDS occurred in individuals employed in health care. Each disease spreads in specific ways, and any therapist who is affected should be educated about the possible risks to others and how to prevent disease transmission.

The ethical dilemma here is whether all information about therapists' conditions and diseases should be disclosed to all clients. Therapists have the right to refuse to treat clients whose conditions present a risk to the therapist. Should clients have the same right—but only if they actually are at risk? Unfortunately, many of these serious diseases have a great stigma attached to them, and the public is scared of what they do not know or understand. For example, HIV is not transmitted by physical contact with the hands, yet some clients may still be fearful of an HIV-positive therapist. Therapists with such a disease may be justifiably afraid of losing clients if they disclose their own health information. Therapists also have a right to privacy.

SCENARIO

Samuel had been practicing massage for 5 years at a very busy resort spa. In this time he built up a regular clientele who often requested him for their vacation massages. Two week ago, Samuel learned from his doctor that he was HIV-positive. Although personally devastated by the news, he was not worried about his massage practice. The doctor reassured him that he would likely not develop AIDS for many years to come and could possibly lead a very normal life for a decade or more. The doctor also gave him information about how HIV is spread and precautions to take. Samuel read all of the information. He knew that HIV is not spread through skin-to-skin contact but understood that he must watch carefully for any breaks in his skin or other ways his body fluids might infect others. Samuel now must decide if he will tell his employers and his clients.

Discuss the following questions, considering each possible action:

1. Should Samuel tell his employers and clients? What are the advantages and disadvantages of telling and not telling?
2. Is there one ethically and professionally correct thing to do?
3. List possible ways Samuel could handle this situation while being ethical and professional.

Realistically, at times you may have a cold or the flu and will need to call your clients to reschedule their appointments. Clients will generally understand that you are not feeling well and will appreciate your not sharing your illness with them. Chronic contagious conditions, however, need to be addressed in a different way. Understanding the risk to your clients is the first step in acting ethically. Check with your health care provider for the most current information to help you make an informed decision about the risk. Will there be a risk to your clients if you follow all precautions? Do any state laws or rules address this issue? (Local ordinances in some areas require therapists to be tested for sexually transmitted diseases.) If there is a potential risk that the disease could spread to clients, how should you inform them of this risk?

These are very difficult questions for a therapist who becomes ill. There are no simple solutions or answers, no one or two rules that apply in all situations, and the ethics of such a situation are not clear-cut. Acting ethically involves research, education, and assistance from other supportive professionals to make an informed choice to ensure the safety of clients. Currently, no laws require health care workers to disclose their personal health history to patients or clients they are treating. Still, a therapist who has a contagious disease should examine all risks for clients. For example, what should a therapist do if diagnosed with hepatitis B? Research shows that hepatitis B is generally spread through body fluids. If this therapist has a cut on the arm, he or she must take all precautions to avoid exposing clients to this area. Talking with one's health care provider also helps one make an informed choice about possible risks to others.

Consider that if you were being treated by a health care professional who had a contagious condition, you would expect that professional to have carefully researched how to protect you from harm. As HIV became widespread, questions of ethical behavior have been carefully studied. Health care providers also have a right to privacy about their health. Overall, again, there are simply no definitive rules regarding disclosing such information to clients. Most professional groups and associations ask health care providers with contagious conditions to become educated about their condition and take precautions to ensure clients are not at risk. In fact, some health care providers have changed to other careers when they felt that their condition did put their clients at risk. In areas where sexually transmitted disease tests are required for licensure, a therapist may be denied a license to practice if found positive.

Key Points

- Therapists should truthfully disclose their credentials and training in techniques.
- Therapists should provide clients with realistic expected outcomes of their treatment.
- Clients expect a therapist to disclose any infectious conditions that could affect them.

DISCLOSING PERSONAL INFORMATION

In addition to health information and information about training and techniques, therapists or clients may intentionally or inadvertently disclose personal information. Several questions may be involved:

1. What information should be considered personal?
2. Who determines if the information is personal?
3. Why is the personal information being disclosed?
4. What responsibilities does the listening party have?
5. When one receives personal information, what should be done with it?

DISCLOSURE BY CLIENT

Any information a client discloses to a therapist may be considered personal information. This includes but is not limited to the information on the health history form and information the client tells the therapist. When the information is relevant to the treatment of the client, this can be considered assessment information. Strictly personal information, in contrast, is not relevant to the treatment that a client is receiving. For example, information about what a client and her friends did last weekend or how a client is treated by a spouse is personal information.

During massage a client and therapist are alone for a period of time. Initially, some clients may talk or disclose information out of nervousness, but as the therapeutic relationship begins to develop, clients often disclose information because they feel comfortable with the therapist and may seek advice. An earlier chapter described how transference can occur when clients looks to the therapist as an important person in their lives. If a therapist reminds a client of a parent figure, for example, the client may look to the therapist for acceptance or advice and may disclose personal information. Many clients also consider their therapist an "expert" in health matters and may disclose information as a part of seeking the therapist's health advice. For example, a client asks for no deep abdominal work because she is having a female reproductive problem. During the session, she talks more about her problem, looking to the therapist for advice about natural remedies for her condition. It is natural to want to help a client and offer advice. A therapist could have had a similar condition or know someone with the same condition. But the therapist needs to maintain professional boundaries and understand that giving advice outside the massage scope of practice is not ethical. Referring the client to another professional is the ethical way to handle this situation. Therapists should help clients understand their scope of practice and knowledge base.

Clients' lives sometimes involve emotional stresses that contribute to physical stress and strain. Massage therapists know that emotions can affect the human body physically. Stress caused by emotional issues and situations can cause a great deal of tension in the body and other physical problems. Many clients seek massage to help relieve them of this tension. But where do we draw the line between what we treat and what we do not treat? Working out tension in muscles is within our scope of practice, but advising clients about dealing with the causes of their stress could easily lead to stepping outside our scope of practice. For example, a client reports that her neck and shoulder pain results from work stresses caused by a boss who treats her unfairly. She wants to talk about her work situation. Working on her tense areas is within the scope of practice of massage therapy, while talking with the client about how to manage her boss is not. Clients can easily take as advice even casual comments from a therapist, but this is beyond the scope of practice for massage therapy.

Bodyworkers have a natural inclination to want to help clients feel better. This attitude may lead to a willingness to listen to clients' problems and other personal information during a session. Clients do want an outlet for their tension. But when is the line crossed? Is just listening to a client going too far and changing the focus of the session? Or is it problematic only when we begin to give advice or offer suggestions? Should bodyworkers discourage clients from even talking about themselves? In their book *The Psychology of the Body*, Elliott Greene and Barbara Goodrich-Dunn explain, "massage may indeed evoke, as a bodily experience that stimulates interaction between the body and mind, elements of the psychological life of the client. However, these elements are the by-products of the massage, rather than the central purpose or focus. Once these by-products become the central purpose or focus of the massage therapist, it is likely that the line has been crossed, and the massage therapist is acting in a psychotherapeutic capacity."

Some bodyworkers feel inclined to give personal advice to their clients, and this is clearly beyond their scope of practice. As massage professionals we need to understand why and how the body reacts physically and emotionally, and know how to assist clients back into a proper therapeutic relationship.

CASE STUDY

Addison received a massage every 6 weeks at her local spa. She felt very comfortable with her therapist. On her way to her appointment this week, she was thinking about the areas that needed attention. Her lower back had been aching over the last couple of weeks. Her therapist, Ron, always asked what areas she wanted to have worked on, and she decided she wanted extra attention given to her lower back today. As Ron was working on her back, she asked him why her back hurt so much. He asked her a few questions about her lifestyle and posture and what had changed in her life in recent weeks. Addison began to tell Ron about her added responsibilities at work and how she disliked that her boss had asked her to do additional work. She began to talk about her boss and asked Ron's advice about what to do at work. Ron realized that even talking about this made Addison's back tighten even more. Ron explained that he could not give advice about what to do at work but continued to work on the physical aspects of her back pain. Ron stayed within his scope of practice while gently guiding the client back to the physical issue of her back.

It is not unusual, when you have had a client for months or years, that you will learn some personal information about them. For example, a weekly client who is getting married soon is stressed out by all the things that she needs to do and talks to her massage therapist about it. Clients frequently give simple information about what is causing their tension. Casual conversation with clients is not unusual. But when conversation starts happening during a session, focus on the treatment is easily lost and clients may not receive what they came for. You can help control a client's talking by keeping conversation light and brief, not asking questions, and bringing the client back to the area you are working on by encouraging breathing and relaxation.

If a client is deeply upset by a situation, a referral to another health care professional such as a psychologist may be appropriate.

DISCLOSURE BY THERAPIST

On the other end of the spectrum are therapists who disclose their own personal problems and information to clients. It is not uncommon to hear clients say their therapist spent the entire hour talking about their lives, relationships, pets, children, etc. Sometimes therapists try to engage the client in conversation by asking about their personal lives. Imagine what a client must feel like when they were only looking forward to an hour of peace but instead have to listen to the therapist talking the entire time? No only would this be frustrating and the client's needs not be met, but it would be unlikely that the client would return for another appointment.

Therapists sometimes act this way in an attempt to fulfill their own personal needs. Something may be lacking in the therapist's life, and the therapist loses sight of the therapeutic relationship. An important ethical boundary involves maintaining a professional and therapeutic relationship that serves the client's needs. A therapist's disclosure of personal information does not serve the needs of the client. A massage therapist who feels the need to disclose personal information while treating clients should seek the assistance of other professionals as to why this is happening.

In some cases a therapist may feel it is showing empathy to the client to disclose personal information that shows the therapist has had an experience similar to the client's. For example, a therapist might say, "I know how you must feel about all that stress caused by your job. When I was in school I worked nights at this busy restaurant and was stressed all the time. . . . " Yet telling the client about this job stress will not help meet the therapeutic goal of relieving physical stresses—if anything, the shift in focus away from the session will reduce the effects of the massage. Therapists can demonstrate empathy for a client's situation or pain without needing to demonstrate it with personal information. Professional boundaries should still be maintained.

Some clients may ask you personal questions. This may simply be the nervous reaction of a client who does not yet feel comfortable with receiving a massage in silence. Friends and family especially will often want to talk during massage. The client may also feel a need to know more about you. New therapists can become really frustrated with such personal questions. You are nervous about performing the massage, and it takes a great deal of concentration to make sure you are doing everything right. If a client

---

BOX 8-2 | *Best-Kept Secrets*

Any time someone is on your table or seeking advice about massage, the therapeutic relationship is in place. The person on the table is your client and you are the therapist. The client deserves to receive a massage with no interruptions. Your client deserves the best that you can give.

Each time I put my hand on the doorknob to enter the therapy room, I stop and take a moment to say to myself, "This person will receive the best massage I have ever given. The person deserves a full hour of my attention and focus on his or her well-being."

---

is asking you questions on top of this, the flow of the session is usually disrupted. Many massage instructors teach students ways to bring the client back to the focus of the session. Once a conversation gets started in a session, however, it can be hard to stop the conversation so that the client is still and enjoys the work that you are doing. You may easily lose your focus and not pay attention to the work that needs to be done.

Boundary issues can arise once a client knows personal information about you. Instead of the therapeutic relationship involving the therapist's focus on the client's well-being, the situation can evolve to the point where the client becomes concerned more about what is happening in the therapist's personal life.

Key Points

- Information disclosed by a client should be used to help assess conditions and plan the treatment.
- A client's personal information should not become part of a session or the therapeutic relationship.
- A therapist's personal information should never be part of a session or the therapeutic relationship.

EXERCISE 8-3

1. Write down the names of five people to whom you have given massages in the past month. Beside each name, list what you talked about other than the client's pain level, comfort level, and sense of being warm or cold.

2. Write down five things you can do to bring a talkative client back to the awareness of the session.

SUMMARY

With all types of disclosure by a client or therapist, there may be times when ethical boundaries are tested. Clients may intentionally or inadvertently raise such issues. Understanding what is ethically right or wrong in the disclosure of information will help you address such situations quickly and without hesitation. Knowing you are doing what is best for your client is a good feeling, leads to clear-cut boundaries, and promotes a good reputation for a successful massage career. Clients will know by your actions that you have a strong foundation in the ethics of disclosure.

ETHICS OF WORKING WITH OTHER PROFESSIONALS

9

CHAPTER PREVIEW

- Awareness of your public image
- Building professional alliances and relationships
- Working ethically with other professionals
- Referrals to and from other health care providers
- Use of consultations
- Team practice issues
- Working in a supervised environment
- Professional courtesy between professionals

KEY TERMS

Consultation: the process of obtaining advice from another professional in the same or related field

Professional courtesy: a professional doing a favor for another professional

Referral: the process of sending a client to another professional for care

Supervision: working under the direction of another professional

Throughout your career as a bodyworker, you will work with a variety of professionals, both in and outside your profession. It is important to understand the complexities of these relationships and how working with other professionals affects your own success. Massage therapy sometimes seems an isolated profession because you are usually working one-on-one with clients. Other professionals, however, can assist you in your growth and success as a practitioner. This chapter will help you understand how to connect with other professionals and how to use these relationships ethically and to your advantage.

BECOMING A PROFESSIONAL

Being a massage therapist involves ethical responsibility. Doctors, nurses, and many other professionals are known by their profession. When they leave work for the day, they do not suddenly stop being a doctor or nurse. Their professional title stays with them 24 hours a day. For example, if you see your health care practitioner at the mall, you most likely first think about him or her as a nurse or doctor, and the fact that he or she is an individual with a life outside the profession is only a secondary thought. This attitude is common about many professions and involves many responsibilities. Your clients and the general public will begin to see you as a massage therapist, even away from work, and your behavior will be scrutinized by others. For example, if you treat a sales clerk in a rude way while shopping and if this person knows you are a massage therapist, he or she may begin to think negatively about massage therapists in general. Lawyers suffer from the image in some people's minds that lawyers are greedy people who are always trying to sue others or make a lot of money. In reality, of course, there are many very good lawyers, who have to suffer from the jokes and stigma of what some people think about lawyers as a whole. Massage therapists have long fought against being associated with the sex trade, but some people still make this association. The example above of a massage therapist treating a sales clerk rudely may seem a rare case, but in fact this can be quite true in small or close-knit communities.

Most owners of businesses that involve customer service will say that they live and breathe their profession. They spend a great deal of time marketing their services and have learned that even one bad situation can hurt business significantly. There is an old saying that people tell only 1 or 2 people about something they like but tell 10 about things they are unhappy about. This can be true of any service profession.

Professionals need to ensure their public behavior is fair and equitable, compassionate, and not sexual or suggestive. Treating all people professionally helps everyone see that you run your business in an appropriate and ethical manner. Avoiding all suggestive or sexual behavior similarly helps others understand that this is not what massage and bodywork are about.

People in all professions and businesses are generally expected to be courteous not only to the public but to other professionals as well. It goes without saying that you should always be courteous to those with whom you are doing business, as well as others in your profession. For example, if other bodyworkers work in your area, you should not try to increase your own business by badmouthing another therapist; the same can always be turned back against you. Someday you may find yourself working side by side with that therapist at a charity event or community function. You may also need to refer clients to another therapist, and having the respect of your peers can work to your advantage.

CASE STUDY

Irene and her friends were having a night out on the town to celebrate her birthday. They tried several locations and stopped at a dance club because things were hopping. Irene had just turned 21, and friends were buying her drinks. After several drinks, her friends got her on the dance floor where they all had a good time, dancing and laughing.

Sitting in the crowd were two couples; one husband and wife were Irene's clients at the spa. Larry and Cindy had been Irene's clients for the last 6 months. They saw Irene on the dance floor and watched the girls having fun, including a little suggestive dancing. The couple they were with asked who they were watching, and Larry and Cindy told them that Irene was their massage therapist. The wife of the other couple said she would never allow her husband to get a massage from someone like that, especially given the way she was dancing. Cindy had never felt jealous or threatened before, but it gave her reason to think about Irene's behavior. She began wondering if her husband now would think of Irene differently while receiving a massage.

Cindy decided to talk to Irene at her next appointment. She told Irene what her friend had said while they were at the club and that it made her worry a little about what her husband might think. Irene was surprised that someone had taken note of her behavior and assured Cindy that she would work in the most professional manner with her husband. Irene had not realized before how her public behavior could affect her professional image.

Once you begin to understand that certain behaviors can be misinterpreted by the general public, you can think more clearly about what you are doing while in public view. Massage and bodywork usually have a very positive image for the public, because the profession helps people in pain and assists in relaxation. But people's opinions can easily change if they see behavior that they do not consider professional. Awareness that your behavior is part of who you are, as is your profession, will help you act in appropriate ways when dealing with others. This does not mean that you constantly have to be on guard or not be yourself; just be aware of the impression you may be making on others.

Key Points
- Take on a professional attitude as you enter the profession.
- Know that the public will be watching you all the time.
- Respect yourself, others, and your profession.

EXERCISE 9-1

Write down examples of five places where you may be seen by the general public, including your clients. For each, list something you might be doing in that place that could give a potentially wrong or hurtful impression to others, which then might affect your career.

Then list ways that you could avoid these types of problems.

PROFESSIONAL RELATIONSHIPS

From the time you first enrolled as a student, you have already been building a network of alliances with other professionals. Whether you decide to work on your own or become an employee in a setting such as a spa, it is important to realize that you will continue to be developing relationships with other professionals.

Your instructors and other students are probably the first people in your growing professional network. Students often seek information from instructors and other students about techniques, skills, and building a business. Because students often have varied backgrounds, it is very possible that people you now know may have been involved with or owned a successful business and can potentially provide you with helpful information to build your own practice. Your instructors and school administrators are also a great source of information to help you become successful. Even while the student–teacher relationship still exists, you should act professionally with your instructors and others in your school. These individuals may soon be making recommendations for you to potential employers and clients. Always acting professionally and taking your education seriously helps you begin to act as a professional bodyworker. For example, if a student is frequently late to class, the instructor may believe that student will also be late for clients. On the other hand, instructors are likely to view a student who is always on time for class and is prepared for assignments as someone who will be successful as a massage therapy professional.

Even while still in school, you are also beginning to develop a network of individuals outside of school who can help you achieve success in the future. Students often report that they have told their friends, family, doctors, local business people, and others about going to school to learn massage. These people may later help you find a location to practice or an employer to work for. Students often report to instructors, for example, that their doctor or chiropractor is interested in learning more about their career and mentioned the possibility of coming to work in their office. Many health care providers also refer their patients for massage, and the professional relationships you begin to develop, even while in school, can lead to business later on. It is good to have other eyes and ears looking out for you and opportunities that may exist.

Professional relationships should always be handled with the utmost of care. As you see in the case of Rachel, you can never know when an opportunity is waiting for you. Developing professional relationships

CASE STUDY

Rachel had become interested in learning more about trigger point therapy. One of her acquaintances, Carole, was also a massage therapist. A day after Rachel had received her monthly massage, Carole told her that she was working for an anesthesiologist in a pain center at the local hospital. Rachel asked what type of work she did, and Carole explained that she did a lot of trigger point work and had trained in myofascial work. Rachel asked if she could observe this type of work before taking classes in this technique. Carole got permission, and the doctor with whom she worked showed Rachel the kind of work they were doing, including their treatment protocols, and explained a great deal about this work. Rachel was thrilled to have spent some time with the doctor and Carole. She wrote letters of thanks to both and then signed up to attend some classes in the techniques they had used.

About a year later, Rachel learned that she would have to close her office because the building was about to undergo redevelopment. She told Carole about it after her monthly session, and 2 days later she received a call from the doctor she had visited at the pain center. The doctor told Rachel she had heard she was closing her practice and referred her to another doctor who was the head of a different pain center. Rachel contacted this other doctor, who, unbeknownst to her, knew about her from the first doctor. The first doctor had been impressed with her when she visited her facility to learn more, and had already given a very strong recommendation to the other doctor. Rachel received a job offer and was thrilled to go to work in one of the most prestigious pain centers in her area.

with anyone you meet can help you in ways that you are yet to realize. Think of each person that you meet as a potential client or a potential connection to a great job opportunity.

You can also deliberately begin to develop professional relationships (Fig. 9-1). For example, if you like the chiropractic office where you have been a patient and would like to build your practice there, you can purposefully begin to develop a professional relationship with the doctor and staff. Such relationships may also involve other health care professionals that you or even your family members have seen. It pays to listen to family members' conversations about their health care providers. Don't be afraid to ask your family and friends who they see and think would be good connections for you to make. You can write a letter

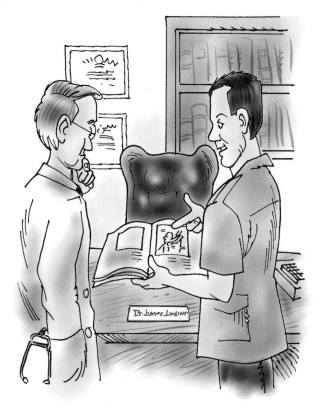

FIGURE 9-1 ■ Developing professional relationships can help massage therapists build their business through referrals, consultations, and additional resources.

of introduction to another professional mentioning the connection you have in the opening to the letter, and this may help you get your foot in the door to begin to develop a professional relationship. For example, you may start a letter saying, "My mother has been your patient for a long time and speaks highly of your treatment and care of patients." The letter may then explain how your treatment philosophy is similar and how you would like to refer your clients to this professional, receive referrals, and possibly consider the person your mentor.

You can also build professional relationships with other people in the business community. When you realize that you need to have some flyers printed to promote your business, for example, you will seek out businesses in your area that provide such services. Talking with other professionals like these not only gives you information about services you may need but also is an opportunity to promote yourself to people who may be looking for your services. For example, while talking with your local newspaper representative about prices for advertising, you may learn that she has been looking for a therapist to work on her lower back. Openness to all opportunities that present themselves is an important key to being successful. Even when you

have a good business plan, be prepared and flexible to accommodate opportunities that may occur at any time.

Networking with other professionals can involve some ethical concerns. Most important, be sure to network only with other business people or professionals who have a good reputation and ethical standing in the community. If you associate with someone who has been the subject of an investigation or who is a subject of gossip in your community, this could cause problems. For example, if you have lunch frequently with the owner of a business that was mentioned in a newspaper article about an insurance fraud investigation, the public might associate you with unethical behavior. If such a person wants to come to you as a client, you have a professional decision to make. Often you can treat clients who do not share your ethical make-up, and in such cases you must maintain a professional demeanor and not become involved in a client's problems. If other clients notice that you are treating that client and raise a question, you can again remain professional and tell them that you do not get involved in people's personal issues when you provide services to clients.

CASE STUDY

At a local auto shop Jonathan was waiting to have his tires rotated when the man next to him started a conversation. Jonathan learned that he owned a large florist shop in town. The man talked about how busy they were with Mother's Day coming up soon and mentioned he would like to show his staff how much he appreciated them with a meaningful gift. Jonathan told him that he had done chair massage for several businesses in town and that the employees really seemed to like it. The florist said that he had seen a magazine article recently about this and that he would check with his staff to see what they thought. He called Jonathan 2 days later and booked him for 2 days to work on his staff during the Mother's Day weekend.

Professional relationships will be a part of your business regardless of the setting you work in. The relationships you build with your clients help set the stage for future relationships you will develop. If your clients see that you handle yourself professionally with them, they will trust you to act in the same appropriate manner with others they refer to you. Because everyone you work on has professional relationships with many others, referrals can involve a vast number of people. Look to every client and everyone you have contact with as having the potential to help you become successful.

Key Points
- Start networking now.
- Every person you meet can be a potential client or a potential source of information.
- Treat others the way you would like to be treated.

ETHICAL BEHAVIOR BETWEEN PROFESSIONALS

Once you realize the potential for developing a professional relationship with everyone you meet, you begin to see the importance of ethical behavior in everything you do. Just as you may make a good impression, the potential is also there to make a bad impression. For example, if you talk about other professionals in a negative manner while you are treating a client, the client is not receiving the best treatment because you are giving a personal opinion. Both clients and potential clients look to you as a health care provider and a bodyworker, someone who nurtures and has compassion. It can be challenging to stay objectively focused in all sessions on the treatment you are providing the client. Clients will ask your opinion about a great variety of subjects beyond the realm of bodywork, including nutrition, fitness, psychological issues, medications, and other health care treatments. Ethically, how should you answer a client without sharing a personal opinion? For example, what should you say if a client asks you about a medical doctor in your area whose treatment you were not pleased with or about whom a client told you about a bad experience? Would you tell the client about your experience or another client's experience? You should think through all the implications before answering such questions. Exercise 9-2 lists questions to explore.

It would be naïve to say that all professionals always act professionally. Many front page stories in recent years have involved ethical issues, and the public is familiar with corporate CEOs and others who have harmed people by behaving unethically. Unfortunately, little is written in most codes of ethics about the ethical behavior that should exist between professionals.

A difficult situation may occur when a client tells you about a type of therapy he or she has received, such as physical therapy, that did not work, or says that the physical therapist was not helpful. It would be dangerous to assume on the basis of this report that all physical therapy or therapists are bad or even that the specific therapist was incompetent. What this simply may mean is that physical therapy was not the best type of work for that client. Treatment is

EXERCISE 9-2

Explore the sample client questions listed below and write out a response to each:

1. What relationship do you currently have with the other professional?

2. Is it within your scope of practice to advise the client about the subject?

3. Could your client be harmed if you did not tell him or her about the subject?

4. What harm could come to you if you give advice?

5. Is your information completely subjective? Should you share that with the client?

similar to medications: some work better for some clients, while others need a different medication. In many cases clients have to try different types of therapy to find the right one for their condition. Massage therapists should think of this as a pathway to their door. If another therapy did not work, the client will seek out alternative therapies, which may include the type of work that you do.

Although clients may want to discuss the failure of other therapies they have tried, it is best not to dwell on such issues when talking with them. You can simply tell the client you are sorry the other therapy did not work but that you will try your best to help them with a different therapy. This approach helps clients consider your therapy more positively rather than focusing on negative or past experiences. Your own comments about the failure of other therapies or therapists would not be helpful to the client and are not appropriate ethically.

It can be difficult at times to avoid sharing your personal opinions. Clients will often ask your opinion about other doctors, therapies, and even other businesses in your community. The ethical approach is to stay neutral. For example, if you received treatment from a chiropractor that you did not particularly like, it may be only your personal opinion that the chiropractor or that particular type of treatment was not what you needed. Yet the treatment that you received may be just the right therapy for your client. If you gave a doctor a massage and the doctor

---

BOX 9-1 | *Best-Kept Secrets*

In cases when another therapy has not worked for a client, do not dwell on this negative reality. Every time another therapy does not work, the client is more likely to find the pathway to your door.

did not like your particular type of work, you would not want the doctor to tell everyone you are not a good therapist. The different types of therapies are options for the public to choose among, and from an ethical standpoint it is best to tell your clients neutrally about the available options and let them choose.

Several guidelines can help you avoid ethical dilemmas and behave ethically as the public has come to expect:

- **Stay within your scope of practice.** Know where your boundaries are as a bodyworker. Staying within your scope of practice prevents giving opinions in areas in which you are not trained. For example, if a client asks you what herbal supplements may help achy muscles, you should refer the person to someone who is trained in nutritional supplements.
- **Stay neutral.** From the client's perspective, your personal opinion will seem a professional opinion. A client who asks you about a type of treatment may give more weight to your opinion than that of someone else who may actually be more knowledgeable.
- **Be sure of your facts.** Giving clients partial information can be dangerous. For example, if you tell clients about nutritional resources, you should also tell them to do more research themselves because you are not an expert in this area.
- **Refer clients to other resources.** Refer your clients to other information sources such as the Internet or library to research a subject.
- **Put yourself in the other person's place.** Think about how you would feel if another professional talked about you in the same way.

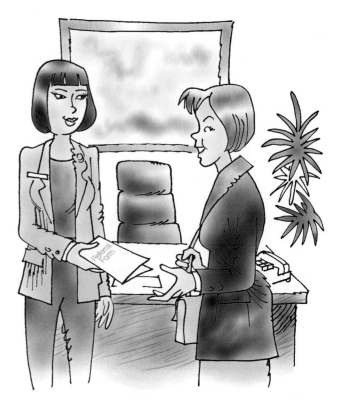

FIGURE 9-2 ■ Referring a client to another health care provider shows your focus on the client's well-being.

> *Key Points*
> - Realize the importance of ethical behavior in everything you do.
> - Clients generally consider your opinion as a professional opinion.
> - Know the boundaries of your scope of practice.

REFERRALS

Referrals can be an important aspect of your business, not only for the number of clients that you may receive, but also in terms of how you take care of clients in an ethical way. Clients want to believe that you have their best interest in mind when you are working with them. If they know that you would refer them to a different therapist for another type of

therapy that would work better for them, they will look at you as a professional (Fig. 9-2). A professional always keeps the client's best interests in the forefront. Unfortunately, a client or patient is sometimes advised to try a type of therapy that may not be best for that client's needs. For example, if a patient is referred for 8 weeks of physical therapy and shows no improvement, it might not be ethical for the doctor to simply continue the physical therapy without considering whether some other therapy might be more effective. Physical therapy produces successful outcomes in most cases, but in some a different type of therapy could have more benefit for the client. Health care professionals should help clients seek out all possible solutions to their problems.

RECEIVING REFERRALS FROM OTHER HEALTH CARE PROVIDERS

Doctors, psychologists, and other health care providers often refer clients for massage when they think it will be beneficial for the client's health and well-being. Developing relationships with health care providers who may refer clients to you may take some effort but can be beneficial for both you and clients. First, referrals are a good source for new clients. Second, when the referring health care provider believes that the client will benefit from the therapy you provide, this is a win/win situation for everyone. Referring health care providers show these clients that they are interested in their well-being, the client benefits from the therapy you provide, and you have a new client. In such cases it is important to maintain good relationships with both the client and the referring health care provider (Box 9-2).

When you receive a referral from another professional, always acknowledge the referral. Referrals may come from other health care providers, and it is important to check in with them about the client. They may have referred the client for specific reasons, and you should know their expectations before you begin treatments. Before any information can be exchanged between two parties about a patient or client, the client must sign a consent form that allows the information to be shared (see Chapter 10). The referring party may want the client to have a certain number of sessions or treatments during a specific period of time. This information helps you formulate an appropriate treatment plan for the client. When the time limit or number of sessions is completed, you refer the client back to the original party who may assess how the client is doing.

If a client asks for a treatment that is different from the treatment specified in the referral, always check with the referring party. It is unethical to give a referred client a type of therapy different from what was originally intended. If you believe that a different approach may be helpful to a client, talk with the referring party about a possible change in treatments to avoid any confusion.

CASE STUDY

Dr. Casey decided that his patient Josh would heal faster from his lower back injury with myofascial release therapy. He referred Josh to Ann, a massage therapist who had treated several of his patients with much success. Ann called his office and faxed a consent form by which Josh gave the doctor permission to tell her about his case. They discussed the need for myofascial release and the areas the doctor thought needed to be covered.

After working on the Josh for several weeks, Ann realized that some other areas too needed attention, but the doctor had not mentioned these in the initial referral. Ann therefore called the doctor and discussed a change in plans before proceeding with Josh's treatment. The doctor appreciated Ann's call and gave his permission for the additional areas. Ann explained the change to Josh, who appreciated the fact that both health care providers were working together to make his condition better.

After the number of sessions had ended, Ann referred Josh back to the doctor and sent a report detailing the work and treatment outcomes.

It is important that both parties in a referral agree on the goals for the client and understand that any changes in the goals or treatment of the client must be discussed with the other party. In some cases a health care professional may refer a client for massage but not specify a particular modality that should be used. Other health care professionals may be very specific. For example, a doctor may refer a client for neuromuscular therapy for 6 weeks to increase the client's range of motion in the neck. If you do not understand what type of work the referring party wants or the outcomes being sought, check in with the referring party to clarify the treatment. If you believe that other types of therapies would benefit the client, it is important to discuss this with the referring party before talking with the client. There may be times when other health care professionals do not know about massage modalities or the benefits they can have for a client. It is important to stay within the guidelines that are given in the referral. It would be unethical to do any type of treatment that was not covered in the referral.

After receiving a referral, it is always good to follow up with the other professional with a thank you note or letter letting the other party know you appreciate the referral. For example, if a chiropractor refers a number of clients to you, it would be good to acknowledge each referral with a thank you note and then possibly a small gift during the holiday season.

FEES FOR REFERRALS

Reimbursements from one professional to another for a referral have long been an issue for health care professionals. Many professionals say this is just a part of doing business, while others feel that fees for referrals are unethical, are actually "kickbacks," and should not be legal. In some states, it is not legal to receive financial gain for referring a client to another health care facility. For example, in some states it is illegal for a doctor to refer patients to a physical therapy facility that he or she owns. In such a case the doctor would make money from both the original visit and the referred physical therapy. Most professional associations do not have clear-cut guidelines about referral fees. It is often up to individuals or businesses to determine what they feel is appropriate and are comfortable with.

Many professionals feel that it is difficult to remain objective when referral fees are given. For example, if you know two dermatologists who treat skin conditions and one offers you a small fee for client referrals, would you be more likely to send your clients to that one? If your clients knew you were receiving a referral fee, would they feel offended or wonder if that is why you referred them? Every individual and business must consider these questions and formulate appropriate policies. Look at both sides of the referral issue when making this decision. Some professionals use referrals to increase their business, and the referral fee is considered a way of saying thank you for the business. For example, a chiropractor may send a restaurant gift certificate to other professionals who refer new patients to them. It is unlikely that other professionals would send new patients to a doctor they considered incompetent just to receive such a gift. The person making the referral is acting ethically in sending a new patient to a doctor who is competent in the appropriate treatment. The referring person simply receives a small token for doing what he or she would have done anyway. On the other hand, if a person sends clients to another health care provider, regardless of whether they need the services, and receives a fee for doing so, many would argue that the referral fee in such cases is unethical.

Referrals between practitioners and health care providers can be a very rewarding experience for clients who receive care from both. Referrals must not, however, involve any conflict of interest. The patient's or client's quality of care should always be foremost. If a therapist is motivated at all by any reason other than the client's well-being when making a referral, the situation should be closely examined. For example, could a sudden unexpected increase in your expenses affect your decision to refer a client to a professional who pays a referral fee? Clients and other professionals would see referrals made for financial or any other reason besides their well-being as improper behavior. One should be careful to avoid even the appearance of impropriety.

Check your state's laws, rules, and regulations, as well as the guidelines of professional associations you belong to, for their policies or information about referral fees. If there are no guidelines, laws, rules, or regulations that apply to you, it is important for you to decide how you will handle this issue. Set your own policy regarding referral fees and be consistent in your business.

REFERRING CLIENTS TO OTHER HEALTH CARE PROVIDERS

It would be wonderful if bodyworkers could provide all the health care services clients need. Obviously, however, some clients will have conditions you are not familiar with or need medical attention or other therapies that you do not perform. Clients may also be seeking a type of massage therapy that you are not trained in. In all such cases, it is appropriate and ethical for you to refer clients to other health care professionals who can provide the appropriate services. It can be difficult to accept that you may lose the clients, especially when you are a new therapist who is still seeking clients. But it is important to consider what is best for the client.

New clients sometimes assume that you know how to treat all muscular conditions and look to you for all services. A client may want a sports massage, for example, but if you are not trained in this technique, you should refer the client to another therapist who does sports massage. Tell the client what types of work you do perform, and explain what outcomes can be expected from that work. If the client chooses your type of therapy and accepts the likely outcome, the client has made an informed choice. But if the client is specifically seeking a type of therapy that you do not perform, or you know a different therapy would be more beneficial, it is best to refer the client to another appropriate professional.

At other times, too, a referral may be appropriate. If a client is very emotional during a session, such as frequently crying, it may be appropriate for you to offer the name of a counselor or psychologist to help the client deal with emotional issues. It is natural for you to want to help the client yourself at an emotional time, but bodyworkers need to remember their boundaries and scope of practice—and that it is not ethical, as tempting as it may be when wanting to help a client, to cross the line into a psychologist's scope of practice. It is appropriate to be supportive of your client through an emotional time, such as explaining that this type of response can be a normal reaction to bodywork. Bodywork can bring buried emotional issues to the surface.

If these issues are troublesome for a client, however, a referral would be in order. Clients will appreciate your concern when you refer them to someone who can help them deal with problematic or painful emotional responses.

PROFESSIONAL ALLIANCES AND ETHICAL BEHAVIOR

It is helpful to begin immediately to develop alliances with other health care providers with whom you can network, refer, and consult in your career. Begin by looking to people you already know, such as your doctor or physical therapist, to whom you can refer clients as appropriate. Research local professionals to whom you can refer clients. Bodyworkers should maintain a resource file with the following:

- Medical doctors
- Specialties such as orthopedic pain centers
- Psychologists or counselors
- Physical or occupational therapists
- Chiropractors
- Other massage therapists that practice other types of modalities
- Crisis centers or support groups
- Clergy

If you do not know anyone in a field, contact professionals practicing in that field and ask them about their services, letting them know you are looking for someone to refer your clients to when appropriate. In turn, they too may be looking for additional resources for their referrals.

If you refer a client to another massage therapist because you cannot provide the appropriate treatment, the client is likely to stay with that therapist. If you refer a client to another health care provider for a specific treatment, however, you can expect to have that client return to you afterwards. For example, if you refer a massage client to a chiropractor for a back injury, when the client is feeling better, the chiropractor should suggest that the client return to you for continued treatment. Unfortunately, not all professionals act ethically to send the client back to the original party. It is also possible that clients may like the person to whom you referred them and may decide to remain with that person for continued treatment. It is important to recognize that clients have the right to choose their treatment.

Working with other providers requires a respect for others and the treatments they provide. Communicating with other health care providers to understand their expectations helps prevent many uncomfortable or unethical situations. For example, if you refer a client to another massage therapist, it

is good to communicate to the other that you are referring the client for a specific number of treatments and then you would like to evaluate how your client is doing at the end of those sessions. If you see that the client is progressing and additional treatments would be helpful, you again should communicate with the other provider. It would be unethical for the other massage therapist to suggest the client have a different treatment protocol without talking with you first.

Always remember that your referred client should not be caught in the middle between providers. For example, if a chiropractor has referred a client to you for neuromuscular therapy for a shoulder injury and you feel that another type of therapy would be more beneficial for the client, you should talk to the referring doctor before discussing it with the client. Telling the client that you would like to switch treatments before talking with the referring person is not ethical. Communicating with the referring professional helps ensure the client's care remains the top priority and helps to build professional alliances. Keeping alliances strong with other health care providers depends on both parties acting ethically with all clients.

Key Points
- Refer your clients when other treatments would be beneficial for them.
- Research resources for referrals for your clients.
- Clients should trust that you have their best interest in mind.

CONSULTATIONS

At times you will need the advice of other professionals to help you with your clients or business. A **consultation** is a means of obtaining information from another professional about a particular subject or client. Usually you consult with those you consider experts in the area in which you are seeking advice. Consulting with others can help you be more successful with your clients and business. For example, if you are wondering how the public in your area is responding to another health care provider's marketing mailer, you could consult with that person to decide if a similar mailing might work for you.

During the consultation process, you receive advice from others. Advice from others regarding your business, techniques, treatments, or conditions can help you expand your capabilities when treating your clients. For example, if a client tells

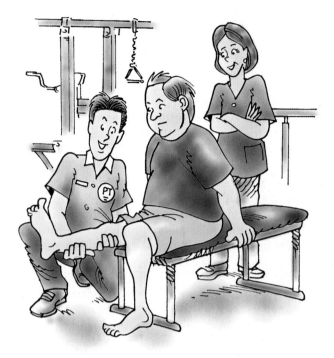

FIGURE 9-3 ■ Consulting with other health care professionals gives you more information to work with.

you about a medical condition he or she has that you are not familiar with, you may consult with a doctor to help you decide whether to treat this client or not. Consultations help to expand your knowledge, which in turn helps your clients (Fig. 9-3). Consulting with professionals you trust can also give you more confidence in your treatment plans.

ETHICAL USE OF CONSULTATIONS

Consulting with others provides you with additional information about a subject, such as a certain condition or type of treatment you are considering using. Other professionals may simply give you advice about how they would treat a client or what they know about a certain condition. There are no guarantees that what they say is correct or the right way to treat your client. Consulting others simply gives you more information to consider. If another professional gives you advice you think is not right or appropriate for your client, you are not obligated to take that advice. In any case, respect the other person for taking the time to give you input on the subject. It is never wise, therefore, to think or speak badly about another person who has given you advice. It is important to maintain a working relationship with others you use as consultants.

Key Points

- Consultations offer more information for a therapist to use.
- Respect the time and effort of the consulting party.
- Seek consultations when you are unclear or unsure about a treatment or condition.

TEAM PRACTICES

Many bodyworkers work in settings where other therapists also practice massage. Several massage therapists may work together as independent contractors in the same office or as employees at a spa (Fig. 9-4). Although the dynamics vary from setting to setting, certain issues are common in these settings.

INDEPENDENT CONTRACTORS

In a setting where everyone works as an independent contractor, each therapist essentially owns his or her own business. It may be as simple as several therapists sharing space in an office or as complex as

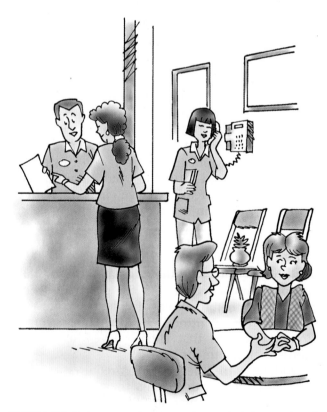

FIGURE 9-4 ■ A massage therapy practice may include a number of therapists working together as a team.

a full facility where one party oversees the general part of the business while everyone still works on their own. In settings where all therapists are their own boss, it can sometimes be challenging for all to agree on issues such as scheduling appointments, hours, advertising, and ethics. The very reason many therapists have their own business is that they like doing things their own way. It is unlikely that everyone will think exactly alike on all issues; often therapists have a wide diversity of opinions about how the business should be run. For example, one therapist may think that a client who does not show up for an appointment should be charged the full amount for the session, while another therapist may not feel it is appropriate to charge the client this way. Chapter 10 discusses how therapists in group practices can work together to establish mutually agreeable policies for an office.

ETHICAL ISSUES IN TEAM PRACTICES

Ethical issues, more than business issues, often seem a stumbling block for therapists in settings where several therapists practice. Therapists often have a wide array of opinions, for example, about socializing with clients. Some therapists have fairly weak boundary lines with their clients, while others maintain a very rigid line. Therapists who have weak boundaries can easily face ethical dilemmas. A client may take advantage of a therapist who lacks a firm foundation, especially when it comes to ethical issues. Other issues too may arise. For example, if one therapist in a practice has a policy that she will never see clients socially and another therapist in the practice does not feel the same, a client who invites everyone in the office to a party may be confused by the different responses from the therapists. It can be almost impossible for a group of independent contractors to agree on all issues they may face. Many successful group practices therefore include only therapists who have similar feelings about issues, or try to reach general agreement regarding ethical issues. At times in a group practice you may have to go about your business and be concerned only with your own practice. Unfortunately, the public views a group practice as one business rather than separate businesses of individuals operating on their own. If a situation occurs that makes you feel uneasy about the ethics of other therapists in a group practice, you may need to find a location better suited to your ethical makeup.

In a practice where one person oversees the business, guidelines are usually set by that person for everyone who practices in that facility. When considering joining a group practice, it is important that you carefully review the members' expectations and consider whether you can follow their policies and guidelines. The practice owner or person who oversees the business wants the public to know what the beliefs and values of the practice are and will ask all therapists to follow and respect the guidelines. Discussing issues with this person will help to prevent complications and resolve any questions you may have.

> *Key Points*
> - Ethical issues versus business issues can be a stumbling block for group practices.
> - A strong foundation can prevent ethical issues from arising.
> - Policies and guidelines can help avoid conflicts.

SUPERVISION

Supervision means that you are working or practicing under the watch of another person or professional. Many therapists work under professionals such as doctors or physical therapists. Supervision is particularly useful when another party such as an insurance company decides that a professional such as a doctor needs to guide the appropriate treatment. Physical therapy assistants, for example, in most cases work under the supervision of a physical therapist. Supervised work does not imply that a therapist is not competent but occurs when another party needs assurance from an experienced or more highly trained professional. Many bodyworkers work under supervision, such as a therapist who works under supervision in a chiropractor's office that bills the client's insurance company.

Working in a supervised environment can be helpful for new therapists. The guidance of another professional can help a therapist formulate treatment plans, help consult about a condition a client may have, and be a source of referrals for a therapist.

In some situations ethical issues may arise in supervised work. For example, a supervisor might ask a therapist to treat a client for 15 minutes but bill the insurance company for 30 minutes. Or a doctor might ask a therapist to bill using a procedure code for a type of work the therapist is not trained in, if the doctor knows the insurance company always pays using that code. Therapists working under the supervision of another professional have been asked to do things that are illegal or unethical. It is very difficult, in such a situation, to question the integrity of an action your supervisor asks you to take. The bottom line, however, is that if you take part in something that you know is illegal or unethical, you are just as guilty as the supervising party. If you participate in a situation that leads to insurance fraud, for example, the authorities will not excuse you because you were working under supervision. You should always understand what is accepted and appropriate in the work you are performing. Don't be afraid to ask questions and seek out answers. In the worst case that may mean that you have to find another person to work under, but even if so, in the long run, you will find it the right thing to do.

Key Points

- Supervision is working under the guidance of another professional.
- Working in a supervised environment can be helpful to a new therapist.
- Having the same ethical policies will help the two parties work more cohesively.
- The ethics of other professionals you work with can affect the public perception of your ethics.

PROFESSIONAL COURTESY

Professional courtesy refers to a professional doing a favor for other professionals. For example, a massage therapist may offer a professional discount to other therapists such as $15 off a session. This is called a professional courtesy because the discount is not offered to the general public. Other types of professional courtesies include making appointments outside normal business hours or offering services that are not generally available to the public, such as payment plans.

Professional courtesies are generally seen as part of doing business and are extended because of advantages for both professionals. Ethical issues seldom occur, although one party may take advantage of another. For example, if a doctor sees another professional during off hours, it would not be ethical for the other professional to expect the doctor to also see their friends and family members during off hours. Taking advantage of another professional can cause bad feelings and result in professional courtesies no longer being extended.

Another type of professional courtesy is one professional offering information that another professional may gain from. For example, if the first professional has heard a complaint from a client about the second professional and knows the client is threatening some type of action, the first professional may pass on information to allow the second to try to intervene and resolve the potential problem. Talking about a client, however, may raise ethical issues of confidentiality.

Professional courtesies often involve decisions for both parties. All services are seldom equal in value. For example, if a massage therapist and psychologist decide to exchange services, the value may not be the same. The massage therapist may normally charge $60 an hour, while the psychologist's fees are $120 an hour. The parties may agree, therefore, to base their exchange of services on the amount of time involved rather than monetary value.

Both parties should be comfortable offering or accepting the professional courtesies. A clear understanding will help prevent conflicts from happening. If either party feels taken advantage of, however, it is important to discuss the issues before the situation gets out of hand. If an ethical issue arises, such as if you feel another is asking you to do something "under the table," a professional courtesy becomes a burden and should be stopped. Professional courtesy in most cases is a good way of doing business and involves effective networking with other professionals.

Courtesy is also good marketing for your practice. Other business owners and professionals appreciate being treated with respect and will in turn be a source of clients or a source for business advice that assists you in your practice. You never know when you may need a favor from someone. Taking advantage of professional courtesies offered to you can be very helpful. For example, if a therapist needs to see a doctor, it is helpful to know a doctor who will make an after-hours appointment on short notice to prevent missing client sessions.

It is appropriate, of course, to reciprocate courtesies that are offered to you. For example, if the doctor who treated you after hours later has a hurt back and needs your services, it is a professional courtesy to fit this person in your schedule as soon as possible.

Key Points

- Professional courtesy is providing favors for other professionals.
- Professional courtesies are services not provided to the general public.
- Professional courtesies should always be reciprocated.

RESOLVING CONFLICTS

Conflicts can happen when you are dealing with other professionals and business owners. You may not agree with the way another professional treats your client, for example, or you may have a personal disagreement with someone.

CASE STUDY

Lindsey had been working in the Sunny Day salon for a year but found the atmosphere was not exactly what she wanted for her practice. Other therapists gossiped about clients and made comments that she frequently thought were not ethical. She decided to move her practice to an office a few blocks away and gave notice to the owner of the spa. The owner was not thrilled because Lindsey had brought many new clients into the spa.

After Lindsey moved, the spa owner, who was also a nail technician, started telling her clients that Lindsey was not a good therapist and making other inappropriate comments. Lindsey heard about this from her clients and decided to speak with the spa owner. The owner denied saying anything, but Lindsey knew better. For Lindsey, this confirmed her move had been the right thing to do. Lindsey in turn decided that she would not speak about the owner or the spa in a negative way. She did not want that type of negative atmosphere in her new place. She spoke again with the spa owner, saying that she would still like to refer clients for the spa's services but that she would have a hard time doing so if negative things were still being said about her. Lindsey told the owner that she would like to part on good terms and even offered to help the owner find someone to take her place at the spa. The owner was surprised and decided to take Lindsey up on her offer and was more careful in what she said to her clients.

Conflicts can involve business matters, such as a problem with your landlord or other tenants in your building or a disagreement with another business in your community. Conflicts can also happen between therapists in the same office. For example, therapists are often upset when one of their clients makes an appointment with another therapist. Although therapists do not "own" their clients, some therapists feel they have a right to clients they have already treated. Another common problem between therapists involves the use of equipment or times scheduled in shared rooms. Quickly resolving such conflicts is important so that clients do not feel the tension when they enter the office.

Conflicts should *never* be resolved through clients. Your clientele should not even know that you are having a conflict with someone else. Clients come to your facility to be treated for their conditions, and involving a client in a conflict is not ethical. Clients often complain that they had to listen to the therapist's issues or complaints during their session. If a client has to listen to you talking about a conflict during a session, the focus on the client's needs has been lost.

Resolving conflicts helps you to stay focused on your work and your clients. There may be times, however, when no matter what you do, a conflict cannot be resolved. In such a case it is still important that your clients are not aware that the conflict even exists. You cannot always change what others say or do, but clients will respect that you have chosen not to involve them in your personal issues. Focus on your client and the session at hand. Deal with any conflicts on your time and in your space.

EXERCISE 9-3

With the class divided in three groups, each group representing a shared business in which therapists practice together and taking one of the examples below, discuss and present to the rest of the class how your group would try to resolve the conflict.

1. The landlord does not want your facility to stay open so late. He has to pay extra for the parking lot lights and security because your office is open later than other businesses in the building. You have 15 regular clients who come during the hours in question.

2. There is a disagreement in your office among several therapists about the days and times that rooms can be used. One of the therapists has been booking clients into another person's time, forcing the other therapist to make clients wait up to 30 minutes. The first therapist refuses to change her appointments because her schedule is full.

3. A therapist in another business located several blocks from your office has been telling people in the community that your business is on the "shady side." A number of your clients have reported this to your office. How can you resolve the conflict with the other business and with the clients who reported this issue to you?

Key Points

■ Conflicts can occur within a practice or with other businesses or people.

■ Client sessions should focus on bodywork and not involve any conflicts.

■ Resolve conflicts as quickly as possible to help keep the focus on your clients.

SUMMARY

Working with other professionals is an important component of a massage therapy practice. Obtaining information, referring clients, and working with other therapists require that you treat others professionally and ethically at all times. Your clients will see that you have their best interests and well-being as the focus of your practice. Treating your clients and others with respect and ethical practices will serve your clients, your community, and your profession.

POLICIES AND PROCEDURES

10

CHAPTER PREVIEW

- Policies and procedures providing the structure and foundation for a therapist's practice
- Values and beliefs helping formulate policy and procedure
- Policies and procedures providing safety for both clients and the therapist

KEY TERMS

Informed consent: a client's right to all pertinent information about a treatment and the granting of permission for a treatment based on that knowledge

Policies: rules and guidelines established for a particular group or population, such as a business

Procedures: processes by which policies and guidelines are carried out

Companies, business owners, and individuals in private practice establish policies and procedures to help their businesses run smoothly, effectively, and ethically. To avoid confusion and inconsistencies, policies and procedures are usually written and collected in a manual. Policies and procedures manuals are living documents that are flexible and can be changed as the business or its needs change. Rules and guidelines help both the business and its clients or customers understand the expectations for the services offered, costs, hours of business, and ethical behavior. The policy manual can be the foundation for a business owner, new employees, and partners to follow. In contrast, businesses without written policies and procedures are often disorganized and experience problems with their clients. Ethical issues can arise. This chapter discusses the importance of policy and procedures for bodyworkers and offers ways to help establish your own guidelines.

WHY POLICIES AND PROCEDURES ARE NEEDED

Policies and **procedures** can form the foundation for your practice and business. Whether you are opening your own business or joining an established

business, it is important to formulate or adopt needed policies and procedures. For example, if you go to work for a spa, you need to follow the policies and procedures established by its owners or managers. These managers set up the policies and procedures to help the business run efficiently and to help clients and employees understand the business and know what is appropriate or not.

At some time you probably have done business with a company or retail store that seemed to lack clear policies or procedures regarding customer relations, such as how to return a purchased item. As a customer you probably felt like its employees did not know what they were doing. Clear policies and procedures, on the other hand, are guidelines that help clients or customers know that the business is concerned with the service it provides and with making its customers as comfortable and as happy as possible.

BUSINESS POLICIES AND PROCEDURES

The guidelines that you set for your business inform your clients and customers of your expectations and what rules they need to follow. For example, you may have a policy that states that all clients have to pay for services immediately following their sessions.

This may seem obvious at first—until you encounter a client who asks to pay after a series of five sessions. Telling this client that your business policy is that all services must be paid immediately after a session and that the business does not maintain accounts-due accounts makes the expectations clear. Without such a policy, for example, the client might not return after a couple of sessions and then you would not be paid for sessions you had already given.

Policies are also needed to prevent situations that you are not comfortable with. If clients see that you have no policy on a specific issue, they may be tempted to try to convince you to do something you are not comfortable doing. For example, a client may pressure you with social invitations if you do not have a policy against not socializing with clients outside the office. Clients and customers expect companies or businesses to have policies and procedures and usually accept them when they are clearly stated or written. Similarly, written policies can help prevent ethical issues from arising with clients. For example, many facilities have a policy that a therapist can refuse service to a client. Quoting the policy is useful if a client makes an inappropriate sexual remark to a therapist. It is not against the law for clients to make sexual remarks, but it is unethical.

It is helpful to have written procedures also for even simple things such as opening and closing the facility. These are particularly helpful for new employees who may need help remembering all the things that should be done at the end of the day (Box 10-1).

Even simple procedures can easily be forgotten, and a checklist in the procedure manual will assist employees who may not normally perform the task. Clear-cut guidelines help prevent problems such as tasks not being completed and having to remind employees what to do.

Once developed, a business's policies should be maintained as consistently as possible for both clients and employees. For example, if a company changes its policy and suddenly no longer accepts checks from clients, customers might become upset. It is important always to inform clients and employees of any changes, therefore avoiding any surprises.

Business policies may include the hours a business keeps, the types of services offered, payment requirements and schedules for clients and therapists, and vacations for employees. Generally two sets of policies are written: one for clients or customers, and a separate policy manual for employees or other individuals working in the office. Policies help support procedures, and vice versa. For example, a group practice may have a policy that payment is required at the end of a session, and the procedure is that the receptionist asks what type of payment the client wishes to make and then writes a receipt for the office records and the client.

PERSONAL POLICIES

Personal policies are guidelines developed by a particular individual in the practice for his or her use. Within a practice of several therapists, different therapists may have different individual policies. For example, one therapist may never work on Sundays, while another keeps this option open. Personal policies too can be written if needed for clear communication to others, or they may simply be orally communicated when needed. Some therapists feel the need to have a written document to confirm their policies when questioned by a client or co-worker or to serve as a reminder. For example, a therapist in a group practice may have a policy that other therapists who use her equipment must sanitize the equipment after each use.

Key Points

- Policies set guidelines for clients and employees to follow.
- Procedures are processes by which policies are followed.
- Policies and procedures should be the foundation of a business.

VALUE OF POLICIES AND PROCEDURES

Policies and procedures help define a business's structure and how it operates. Most people have worked for a company with a policy or procedure manual. When questions arose, answers could usually be found in the manual. For example, if an employee needed to know when the company closed for holidays, the policy manual would answer

---

BOX 10-1 | *Sample Facility Closing Procedures*

1. Turn off all equipment in the laundry area (hot packs, oil warmers, and facility stereo).
2. Check each massage room for any additional laundry and place in laundry room.
3. Empty trash in all massage rooms.
4. Pick up magazines and empty trash in reception area.
5. Lock the back door and deadbolt from inside.
6. Turn off all lights except the front hall light.
7. Put up the closed sign.
8. Lock and double-check the lock on your way out.

that question. Employee policy manuals also can contain information about hiring requirements, expected behaviors and the consequences for inappropriate behavior, management structure, and training agendas. The value of a policy and procedure manual comes in the use of and follow-through with the information the manual contains.

VALUE FOR THERAPISTS

Policies and procedures provide a structure for therapists to use and also help portray a professional image to the public. It can be overwhelming for a person who provides bodywork sessions to also tend to the day-to-day operations of owning or being a part of a business. Structuring daily operations in procedures can help prevent having to make constant decisions about the business and operations.

A business without a clear structure is often in a constant state of chaos and change. For example, if a massage office had no policy about its hours of operation, it would be hard for therapists to set up consistent hours for their schedule and their clients. Successful businesses understand the importance of structure for both staff and customers.

Structure and policy can also help therapists set up their schedules and goals. For example, a therapist who wants to attend 20 hours of continuing education every year needs to begin to schedule time away from the business long before the appointment book becomes full and cancellations would be required. Clients who book on a regular basis can be rebooked ahead of schedule to prevent any problems. If a therapist has a set schedule, it is much easier to make plans and be organized with tasks that need to be completed. For example, a therapist who begins sessions at 9:00 A.M. every day of the week except Wednesday will find it easy to use that time to go to the bank, pick up supplies, and run errands needed for the business. Without a set schedule, fitting in all the detail work becomes challenging.

Policies and procedures can also help a business or individual present a positive, professional image to the public. When providing services to the public, a business is under the constant scrutiny of its customers, particularly its new and potential customers. A potential customer who stops by a massage office to make an appointment and finds inconsistent hours may look elsewhere for services. The public expects and relies on service businesses to have consistency, which results in part from policies and procedures.

A therapist's polices should also help clients understand what services the business provides (Fig. 10-1). For example, a therapist's brochure may

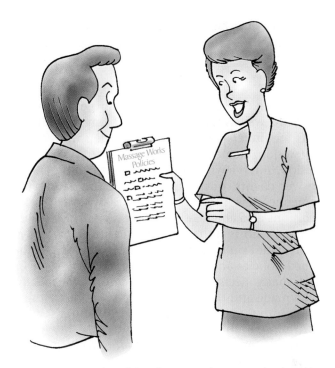

FIGURE 10-1 ■ The policies of a massage therapy practice should be communicated to clients.

state that practice offers sports massage, reflexology, and deep tissue massages. If a client asks for a type of therapy that is not offered, the therapist should have a policy for making a referral for other types of therapy.

Policies also prevent therapists from being put in awkward situations in which they would have to decide on a case-by-case basis what action to take. Not being prepared with an existing policy makes a therapist vulnerable, and a client may try to take advantage of the situation. For example, if a client is 30 minutes late for an appointment and there is no stated policy referring to this situation, the client may still expect to receive a full hour massage, even though that would cause delays for all following clients. But if the therapist has a clearly stated policy that sessions are booked for the designated time only, clients who are late will know that their session length will be affected. This is a good example of a needed policy for practices that need to run on time.

Procedures similarly help provide structure needed in businesses. Procedures for banking, purchasing supplies, and other daily functions help therapists be more organized and plan for the future growth of the business. For example, if you always plan to purchase supplies at the end of the month, you can budget for those supplies during the preceding weeks.

New therapists who think about their policies and procedures being a foundation for their practice have made a good start for handling the often complex issues faced by both owners of businesses and employees working for someone else.

VALUE FOR EMPLOYEES

Policies and procedures help employees in much the same way as business owners. Many new therapists are understandably nervous when they begin a new job. Remembering what to do during the session, interviewing the client, and being able to answer clients' questions can be intimidating for someone new in the business. Having to make decisions also about issues such as what to do with a client who is unhappy with service or has payment issues only adds to that nervousness. Established policies and procedures for employees mean that many decisions such as these have already been made and the employee can more easily transition into the business.

An important educational aspect of being an employee involves learning an employer's policies and procedures. Often policies are set by business owners or managers who are not bodyworkers, and sometimes it is difficult to put these policies into play. For example, many spas schedule appointments only 15 minutes apart. Depending on the spa's physical setup and the availability of help from other employees, this policy may not be practical. If the therapist also has to check the client out, take payment, book the next appointment, and prepare the room for the next appointment, as well as possibly needing a quick moment alone to refresh, 15 minutes may not be enough time. Seeing what works or does not work also helps new therapists understand what they may want to do if they set up their own business. Therapists who choose to stay within the spa can help the managers and staff understand the needs of massage therapists in order to better serve clients. Before making or suggesting changes in policies and procedures, however, it is important to understand the employer's original reasons for setting policies and procedures affecting bodyworkers and their clients (Fig. 10-2).

VALUE FOR CLIENTS

Policies and procedures state guidelines for clients and help them know what to expect from a bodywork practice. Many therapists put their office policies in writing, and many require clients to sign a statement that they have read those policies. For example, many massage practices have a policy that states they have the right to refuse service to clients. Such a policy is usually designed to avoid clients who have made inappropriate comments or

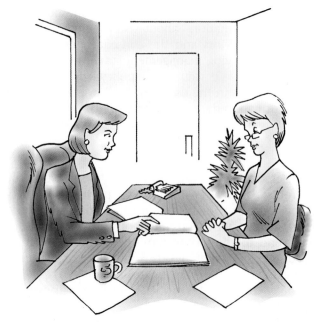

FIGURE 10-2 ■ When you interview with a prospective employer, be sure to learn the employer's policies and procedures.

gestures toward a therapist in the past. Another policy may be that only 1-hour sessions are scheduled. Clients frequently ask for longer sessions, but this policy would let clients know this service is not offered.

Many other policies are designed to help a client feel safe in the massage environment. Policies concerning draping and attending to the client's comfort levels based on the client's feedback are designed to help clients feel more comfortable. The safety and comfort for all parties should also be foremost in the policies of any business.

> ### Key Points
> - Policies are the structure and foundation for practice.
> - Procedures define how policies are carried out.
> - Policies and procedures help protect the safety and well-being of both clients and therapists.

FOUNDATION FOR AN ETHICAL PRACTICE

Beginning with your first day as a massage student, you have been building the foundation for your massage practice. When students first enroll in their massage program, most are not thinking about the many dynamics that will be involved in massage practice, such as emotional issues and responses to bodywork or the marketing of a massage practice. Determining the image to project to the public and the type of work to perform are among the many variables that can set a practice up for success or failure. Many of the other issues discussed in previous chapters can help you understand the importance of the foundation you are building for practice. Therapists who do not believe a foundation is needed and who do not plan for their career, on the other hand, can end up in uncomfortable ethical situations.

Therapists first beginning practice often experience common fears and nervousness. Some clients may sense that nervousness and try to take advantage of a new therapist. For example, if a client tells a new therapist that he or she has never been draped for massages in the past, the therapist may feel obligated to do the same. If a therapist is caught off guard by such a request and does not have a stated policy about draping, it may be hard to tell the client that this is not acceptable. But if the therapist has a policy that states that all clients will be fully draped except for the area being worked on, this makes it easy to tell clients that this is required. The client then clearly knows the expectations for the session.

Just as some clients may "test" a new therapist, in other situations a client may make a request that the therapist simply has not yet thought about. For example, a 13-year-old may request a massage. Most facilities require that a parent sign consent or be present during the session with someone this age. Initially a facility may not have a policy regarding minors, but after experiencing the situation it then sees the need for such a policy. Such problems can be avoided by taking the time, before beginning practice, to consider anything that could happen between a client and therapist and to design policies to prevent or handle such situations. Policies and procedures must be flexible to change when needed, however.

THERAPISTS' INDIVIDUAL BELIEFS AND VALUES

Working in a business with other therapists frequently leads to differences of opinion regarding the ethics of bodywork. As discussed in Chapter 2, one's values and beliefs originate in personal background and upbringing, so it is only normal that therapists will encounter others who have a completely different outlook on some ethical principles involved in bodywork.

CASE STUDY

Lindsey was excited to be hired by a nearby resort spa. During her initial training at the spa, she learned that 15 other massage therapists also worked at the spa, which had developed a considerable business. About half of these therapists worked part time, the others full time. Lindsey was a bit disappointed that she received only a half day of training before beginning to perform massages the next day. The manager talked about routine matters such as laundry, supplies, appointment times, and uniforms. When Lindsey asked about what to do if a client had a problem, the manager was vague and did not answer her questions.

Later, Lindsey talked with two other therapists in the break room and said she was a bit nervous about interacting with clients. She asked them if they had ever had problems with clients who asked them to do something inappropriate. Both of the therapists said it had happened to them, but their responses were very different. One said that she let clients have what they wanted, in this case, to receive a massage without draping. The other therapist told the client that it was her policy that all clients will be draped. A client had tried to talk her out of it, but she told him that if he did not accept this policy, the session would end. Lindsey asked if the spa had policies that addressed these concerns. The other therapists told Lindsey they were not aware of any particular policies and they just handled problems on their own.

CONFLICTS IN BELIEFS AND VALUES

Working for another party rather than for oneself can involve a number of ethical issues. The business may have policies that address issues a new therapist may not have thought about, but also disagreements may arise about policies. Situations may occur in which one's personal beliefs and values are tested. For the sake of a job, should therapists put their own personal beliefs and values aside? This problem is not unique to the bodywork profession but occurs also in many other professions. For example, a business may have a policy about not giving customers certain information before they purchase a product; in this case employees would need to decide whether they want to work for that company if they believe that customers should have all information upfront.

Employees often do not agree with every policy of a business. Employees may disagree with policies involving vacation days, sick days, scheduling, and pay periods when they are required to follow those policies. Policies concerning more subjective issues are more likely to result in a wide variety of opinions among therapists. For example, a business may have a policy that a client will be red-flagged for asking for something sexual yet will book the client again with another therapist. Some therapists would disagree with this policy, believing that this client should not receive services again from the business. Yet another therapist may not have the same problem with the client. Bodyworkers have a great variety of opinions about situations like these. It is important to come to an agreement, in all group practices, about what will be done when a therapist does not feel comfortable working with a client. Being supportive of others and their opinions is an important part of having a successful business.

It is difficult to know in advance, however, all situations therapists may encounter in a business. Therefore, it is difficult to create policies in advance that will cover every possible situation. It is helpful to talk with a mentor or others who have bodywork businesses to learn what policies to consider and even how to make decisions about them.

It is also important to ensure your policies are consistent with state laws, rules, and regulations. For example, if a state rule requires certain parts of the body to be draped during a massage, your policy should be at least as stringent, although it can be stricter if you prefer. If a client questions your policy, you can say that it is both your policy and a state rule that draping must cover certain areas of the body.

Policies can also help you preserve boundaries that will sometimes be needed with clients. A client who does not agree with one of your policies such as draping may choose to go elsewhere. An important question to consider, in such cases, is whether you would feel uncomfortable forgoing the policy. What if that policy is intended for the safety of the client and the therapist?

Ideally, all massage practices should have clear, written policies and procedures, including both independent and group practices and all other businesses. The foundation provided by policies helps everyone know the expectations of the practice. The safety of the client and the therapist should always be foremost when policies and procedures are developed.

Key Points

- Clients will test policies and procedures.
- Diversity in values and beliefs leads to differences in policies and procedures.
- Group practices require compromise and consensus.

WRITING YOUR OWN POLICIES AND PROCEDURES

The process of developing policies and procedures begins with making an initial plan for the business. Initially it is difficult to cover all the areas that need to be addressed. Policy and procedures documents are living documents, meaning they are flexible and should be changed if new issues arise or a policy is not working well.

DECIDING WHAT IS IMPORTANT

Consider two questions when developing policies and procedures:

- "How does this policy or procedure help my clients?"
- "How does this policy or procedure help me?"

Policies and procedures ideally should be helpful to all parties, although some policies or procedures refer to only the therapist or client. For example, a business procedure for making a bank deposit every night involves only the therapist. A policy that requires all clients to have an interview with the therapist before receiving a bodywork session benefits the client by focusing on the health and goals of the client, but it also benefits the therapist by helping give direction to the massage session.

Policies and procedures should also be practical and convenient for the parties affected. For example, if a business makes a policy to accept only cash, this could cause a hardship for clients who rarely carry cash and who show up for an appointment without enough money to pay for the session. Would you send a client to an ATM to get more cash, reschedule the client's appointment, or accept the client's check for that session? All policies and procedures are developed to help a business run smoothly and to provide clients with a quality service. If a policy or procedure gets in the way of that service, it should be revised. Policies and procedures should also be flexible enough that they can be adjusted if they are causing a hardship for one of the parties involved.

Exercise 10-1 helps you identify areas to address when writing your own policies and procedures. As Exercise 10-1 shows, policies and procedures are needed in many areas for a massage business or therapists working as employees. A therapist's own policies may help that therapist have a more successful practice than others in the area. Policies and procedures help motivate the discipline that is sometimes needed to stay focused on the business side of massage.

The MassageWorks sample policies shown in Box 10-3 are just a beginning of a full set of policies

EXERCISE 10-1

For each of the practice issues below, write one or two sentences that state a policy for a massage therapy practice. Try to keep your statements general enough to apply in all or most circumstances.

Example: MassageWorks (business name) will accept clients from advertising, word of mouth, and referral. MassageWorks reserves the right to refuse service to clients who behave inappropriately.

1. Client interview: _____

2. Modalities practiced: _____

3. Draping: _____

4. Acceptable types of payment: _____

5. Referrals: _____

6. Hours of operation: _____

7. Therapists' qualifications: _____

8. Advertising: _____

9. Rotations: _____

10. Seniority: _____

BOX 10-2 *Best-Kept Secrets*

Many successful therapists make it a personal policy to come to work always when scheduled, even if they have no appointments. They can use this time to make reminder calls and follow-up calls, develop marketing plans, and handle phone calls and potential walk-ins. It would be easy just to take the time off when one has no appointments, but having a good work ethic helps a therapist become successful.

BOX 10-3 *MassageWorks Policies (Sample)*

Hours of Operation: MassageWorks is open Monday through Friday from 10:00 A.M. to 7:00 P.M. Appointments are suggested but not required. The last appointment for massage services will be at 6:30 P.M.

Seniority: Therapists who have been with the spa the longest have first choice of days and shifts.

Saturdays: All therapists are required to work at least one Saturday per month.

Schedule Changes: Therapists may not switch shifts with other therapists because many clients make their appointments with a particular therapist. All schedules must be approved by the spa manager.

Draping: Draping clients must follow the strict guidelines in state rules and regulations. Clients who request little or no draping will be told the state rules and the spa's policy. Any therapist who does not drape all clients appropriately is subject to suspension or termination.

therapists should develop for their practices. As you begin your own practice, you will see a need for additional policies and procedures (Box 10-4). Any time you experience a problematic situation, stop to think about how a policy might have prevented or solved it. Then write a policy to prevent or solve similar problems in the future.

DEVELOPING A MANUAL

Exercise 10-2 along with other suggestions made in this chapter can help you formulate the beginning of a policy and procedure manual for a new massage or bodywork business.

As you write your policies and procedures, think about how to best present them with a professional appearance. A few notes handwritten in a notebook are a beginning, but a neatly word-processed or typed format will look more organized and professional when you show it to others who may be considering working with you in a facility (Fig. 10-3). Think about what you yourself would expect to see when applying for a position at a business. A professional appearance says a great deal about those looking for quality employees and independent contractors. Think also about how written policies can be presented professionally to your clients, as discussed in the next section.

In a practice in which several therapists work together as independent contractors, policies and procedures may be developed by the group. In any group decision, compromises on issues are sometimes needed. Very rarely does a group of people

**MassageWorks
Policy and Procedure Manual**

Table of Contents

Section III. A.   Hiring Policies   12

MassageWorks' hiring policies will always follow local, county, and state guidelines for massage therapists. These include, but are not limited to, state requirements for all massage therapists to have attended an accredited school, to have a minimum of 500 hours of education, and to have passed the National Certification Examination for Therapeutic Massage and Bodywork (NCBTMB).

County ordinances also include a health screening by a licensed physician, which must be provided to MassageWorks before official hiring can take place. The state requires that all massage therapists carry professional liability insurance, and MassageWorks must retain a copy of the insurance certificate. Professional liability insurance must be kept current at all times. If a therapist does not renew this liability insurance on or before its expiration date, MassageWorks must terminate the employee until the liability insurance has been updated.

New employees are considered to be on probation for the first 90 days of employment. During this time, employees are scheduled for the shifts that have been agreed upon and are expected to fulfill the requirements for working those shifts. If a problem arises with scheduling, the employee should discuss it with his or her immediate supervisor to find a possible alternative. New employees may not on their own ask other therapists to cover their shifts during this 90-day probation period.

Massage therapists must also provide MassageWorks with an original copy of their state license along with a 2x3 current photograph. The license will be displayed in the main office as required by state law. Photocopies are not permitted. Please contact the state board to obtain an original copy. The fee is $5. All original licenses must be posted within 10 days of employment by MassageWorks. If an employee quits or is terminated, MassageWorks will return the license to the employee.

All employees are expected to read and follow the policies in this MassageWorks Policy and Procedure Manual. A copy will be given to all employees on their first day of employment. New employees must

FIGURE 10-3 ■ Give your policy manual a professional appearance.

BOX 10-4   *Other Topics Included in Policy Manuals*

1. Client privacy and confidentiality
2. City ordinances and state law compliance
3. Health and fire department compliance
4. Informed consent
5. Therapists' or clients' right to refuse services
6. Payment for missed appointments or late arrivals
7. Time of payment
8. Socializing with clients
9. Working with friends and family members
10. Insurance reimbursement
11. Referral sources
12. Note-taking and filing procedures

Key Points

■ Look at policies and procedures used in other businesses.
■ Always ask two questions:
  – How does this serve the client?
  – How does this serve the therapist?
■ Consider the well-being and safety of both the client and the therapist.

---

agree completely on every issue. Group work meetings help set the tone for developing a working manual with everyone involved. If one person does all the writing, in contrast, it may be hard for the others to take ownership and pride in what has been written. But if all parties involved bring their ideas and each has a forum to talk about what he or she feels is needed, this approach encourages communication so that the group develops a plan that everyone can work with. If a consensus cannot be reached on important policies, an objective outside resource such as a mentor or consultant can help the group decide the most acceptable compromise.

EXERCISE 10-2

Imagine that you are new owner of a massage therapy practice where four other therapists will work as independent contractors. If possible, look at another company's policies and procedures manual to get a general idea of what areas are covered and the kinds of wording used. Ask your friends, parents, or a mentor if they have a policy manual where they work. Check your own workplace for a manual. All of these can give you good ideas for policies and procedures. Then address these questions:

1. List areas the manual should address.

2. Write a one- or two-sentence policy statement for each area you identify.

3. What procedures should be developed for this new business? Consider what procedures should apply to all the therapists working in this facility.

4. Exchange your policies and procedures list with other students in the class, and give each other feedback.

COMMUNICATING YOUR POLICIES

INFORMING THE PUBLIC

Policies can be conveyed to the general public and to clients in a number of ways. Initially, the first contact with a potential client may involve some discussion about the business's policies. For example, if a new client makes an appointment with you for next week, after confirming the date and time, you may tell the client that you have a 24-hour cancellation policy that requests clients to call in to cancel or reschedule at least 24 hours in advance or they will be charged for the session. Clients then know that they need to call ahead if they cannot make their appointment. Many businesses have this policy, and most will waive the policy in some unavoidable events such as a client who is required to stay late at work or has to care for a suddenly ill child.

Brochures and marketing pieces can also convey a business's policies. The operating hours, types of services offered, and types of payment accepted are important information for potential new clients. Obviously, you need not include here your business policies that do not apply to clients. Other policies can be communicated to clients only as needed. For example, if you require a signed consent form before rendering services, you can state this policy on the intake form. Policies should be written in clear and concise language without sounding harsh (Exercise 10-3).

Informed consent is also a means of providing information to clients. When clients are going

EXERCISE 10-3

Look back over the policies you wrote in Exercises 10-1 and 10-2 and determine if the statements are clear. Ask several other students to look over what you wrote and point out anything that does not seem clear or that seems expressed in negative language.

to receive a massage or therapy, it is advisable to inform them about the type of treatment they are going to receive and the outcome they should expect. Often clients ask questions to help them fully understand the treatment they will have. Most facilities require clients to sign an informed consent form, which states they have been told about the treatment and they consent to it. Generally all health care facilities require that a patient or client sign such a form before any treatments are given.

Informed consent helps both the client and the therapist understand what the session will be about. For example, if a client does not want to agree to a particular aspect of a session, such as energy work, this should be noted and signed by the client and therapist. Ethically, the therapist must be honest about the expected results of a massage treatment; for example, the therapist should not mislead the client to think a pain will be completely gone if the client's condition is such that it may not. Nor should the therapist allow the client to have unrealistic expectations, even if the therapist said nothing to promote those expectations. For example, if a client happens to mention that he or she hopes to never again have a back problem while receiving regular massage, the therapist must correct such unrealistic expectations. Complete honesty is the ethical key to giving information so that the client can give informed consent.

INFORMING EMPLOYEES

When employers and potential employees talk about employment, policies and procedures are generally a major part of the discussion. Both parties need to feel the policies and procedures are workable. During the interview an applicant should ask questions in order to fully understand the employer's expectations of employees. Often a copy of the business's policy manual is given to an applicant to read before accepting the position. If you are considering a position offered to you and you have not seen the policy manual, ask to read it so that you are sure that you can work within the business's guidelines. Sometimes a new employee is very excited about getting a job and realizes only later that he or she is not comfortable with some of the policies. You can also talk with others who have worked or are not working at this business to learn about the effectiveness of the policies and procedures.

From the employer's point of view, it is also better to ensure that potential employees or independent contractors understand all the expectations from the beginning. Preventing future misunderstandings and problems can save a great deal of time and energy.

For example, if a business requires all therapists to work at least two Saturdays a month and an applicant does not want to work weekends, it is better to know this before the person is hired and both parties later discover that it is not going to work out. The more information that can be presented in the preliminary stages, the lower is the risk for misunderstandings and problems.

Once an applicant has accepted a position, it is important that the new employee is trained in every respect. Simply handing an employee a manual and asking him or her to read the material is not enough. There is too much room for interpretation, and questions often go unanswered. Discussing policies in person will help the new employee more fully understand what all policies mean. After being trained, employees should sign a statement saying they have read the manual and have been trained in all policies. This can be helpful for the employer later on if problems develop because an employee is not following a policy.

INFORMING OTHER THERAPISTS

As either an employee or an independent practitioner, it is important for you to inform other therapists and professionals about your policies and procedures and to learn about the policies of other professionals with whom you work. For example, if you refer clients to a certain chiropractic specialist, it would be important to know if this chiropractor's patients are required to see his or her massage therapist while receiving chiropractic care. Likewise, it is important to inform other professionals about any policies you may have that affect clients who are referred to you. The information is best provided in writing so that it remains available to the professional and his or her staff. Many therapists who often use a referral network give packets of information to the referring parties. This may contain promotional material, business cards, and referral policies for staff and potential clients. This can also be an additional marketing opportunity.

> **Key Points**
>
> Policies can be conveyed to others:
> - Verbally
> - By brochures
> - Through signed intake or consent forms

SUMMARY

Policies and procedures form the foundation and structure for most businesses. The policies of a massage therapy practice should be based on offering quality services and looking out for the safety and well-being of both the client and the therapist. The success of the business is often determined by how well policies and procedures are developed and followed. Writing policies should be an ongoing, flexible process. Clearly written policies, when communicated well to clients, help ensure clients that they will be treated fairly and ethically. Similarly, clear communication of a practice's policies to employees and other therapists and professionals also helps prevent problems that might otherwise occur.

BUSINESS ETHICS

11

CHAPTER PREVIEW

- The public perception of ethical business practices as key to success
- Effect of the ethics of others on your reputation
- Effect of your ethics on the business of others
- Ethical responsibilities of owning a business
- Ethical marketing practices that enhance success
- Financial issues that involve ethical responsibilities

KEY TERMS

Independent contractor: a non-employee who provides services within a business

Sole proprietor: a person who owns and operates his or her own business and often works alone

Ethical issues are an important aspect of the business of massage therapy. Business ethics are important both inside and outside the treatment room, and poor ethical practices can easily lead to the downfall of a business. As discussed in previous chapters, when you begin practicing, you become a bodyworker rather than just an individual, and good business ethics is part of that persona. This chapter will help you understand how and why business ethics is an important component of a successful practice.

IMPORTANCE OF GOOD BUSINESS ETHICS

It has been said the public is always watching. Although you may feel your private time is strictly yours, it is a good to remember that whenever you are out in public, someone else could be judging your behavior. For example, if you make a purchase and the clerk gives you too much change, do you keep the extra money or do you give it back? What will that person think of you when he or she realizes the mistake and knows you kept the money? If you gave your own client too much change, wouldn't you appreciate a customer returning it to you? When you stand in the shoes of the other party, would you act or react differently?

The public views businesses in many ways, particularly in the bodywork profession. The business has a financial side involving advertising, money issues, and booking appointments. On the other side is the practice of massage and the public's perception of the actual bodywork being performed. Any public skepticism can easily affect either side. For example, potential clients who feel that a business's advertising is suggestive will assume that the whole business is unethical. Or clients who feel that they did not receive the full hour and a half they paid for may believe the whole practice has poor standards.

It is important for a business to be very clear about its services. It is equally important to also know the client's expectations. If clients pay for an hour and a half, will they truly receive 90 minutes of bodywork? Or is the intake time and dressing time included in that time period? Informing clients about the small details can make a very big difference in how they act or react when an issue arises.

123

A client who knows upfront that an hour session actually means 50 minutes of bodywork will not feel short changed when receiving services.

A business person should always be aware how the business is perceived by clients and the general public. It is a good idea to put yourself in the other person's shoes to see how a policy or procedure would feel if it affected you. Your ethical behavior will affect how people perceive your business. Educating and informing clients can be an important way to prevent problems from occurring and will help clients have a good perception of the services that you provide.

THE PUBLIC'S PERCEPTIONS

News stories often inform the public of wrongdoing by the managers or owners of large companies. Many end up in court for their offenses. Law enforcement agencies determine when a business has committed illegal acts. Unethical acts, even when not illegal, are just as important. A person who feels unfairly treated may file a lawsuit. Even if no legal action is taken, if people feel they have been treated unfairly in some way by a business, this affects their perception of the business. An individual tells other people, and the word spreads. When the public perceives that a business has treated someone unfairly or has done something inappropriate, the public may no longer seek that business's services. For example, if a client has seen a therapist for a series of sessions but still feels the initial problem has not been addressed, this client may tell others the therapist does not give effective therapy. This is another reason it is so important to know clients' expectations and to stay in constant communication to know what they are feeling and whether you and the client are on the same track. From an ethical standpoint, if a client feels that a therapist said something unprofessional, this too can affect the client's and general public's perception of the business. It is very important to weigh your words and actions when working with clients in the bodywork profession.

Bodyworkers, like any other business people, need to maintain good business ethics. But in addition bodyworkers are also still fighting to correct the past perception of massage as a front for illegal trade. Business ethics in massage, therefore, are doubly important. Fortunately, businesses can change the public's perceptions. Educating the public is part of marketing in every business and is one of the most important components of business for bodyworkers. The wording and graphics used in advertising, for example, can easily lead the public to believe a bodyworker is legitimate. While a business name of "Scandals Bodywork" would likely make the public wonder about its services, a business name such as Therapeutic Bodywork gives a completely different impression. Changing someone's perception may mean you gain a new client, who also helps spread the word about your business.

You cannot change the perceptions of everyone you come in contact with, however. People always have their own values and beliefs, as discussed in previous chapters. Not everyone can be convinced that bodywork is a viable, positive kind of work. But the media as a whole have helped the public see what massage and bodywork are all about. Positive news stories are aired more frequently about the value of massage and it is becoming increasingly rare to hear about raids on businesses doing something illegal under the name of massage.

As the public better understands the positive side of massage, bodyworkers can spend less time trying to change the public perception of massage, but we still must deal individually with the business ethics of our work. Handling a business and acting ethically toward others is just as important as, and in some cases can be even more important than, the massage work itself. For example, a great massage therapist may talk to a friend about a client's health, which is a breach of a client's confidentiality. If this friend mentions it to others and it eventually gets back to the client, the therapist certainly will have lost a client. In addition, others who hear the story may feel the therapist cannot be trusted to maintain confidentiality and therefore may not recommend this therapist, resulting in potentially several other lost clients. Some states, moreover, have rules about client confidentiality, so the therapist may have acted illegally as well as unethically. In either case, a wrong has been done to a client, and this is not good advertising for the therapist's business. Another example of poor business ethics is a therapist who tells clients about personal problems during a session. Although some clients may appear not to be bothered by this type of conversation, it is a frequent complaint of clients that their therapists spent much of a session talking about themselves. Clients pay for their sessions to have their own needs met. Listening to someone else's problems is not part of their plan. Frequently, this situation leads to a client not returning to the therapist and not recommending the therapist to others. Many therapists hear such complaints from clients about other therapists.

Bad news travels fast, and unfortunately people like to talk about negative things. If a business gives poor service or has poor ethics, it can be an easy target for the public. The daily news generally emphasizes negative events, and unfortunately the public loves to hear bad news. By paying close attention to public opinions, however, a therapist can build a strong ethical business where clients will feel safe and which they will recommend to others.

> ### Key Points
> - A business that provides service to the public should always be aware of the impression it makes on others.
> - Unethical behavior may or may not also be illegal behavior.
> - Good business and personal ethics help make clients feel safe.

PROTECTION OF THE THERAPIST

Unethical business practices are a direct reflection of the owner and employees of a business. If an individual works in a business that is perceived as having done something unethical, that individual too could be perceived as unethical, even if he or she was not a part of the act. This is why it is very important for both the owners of a business and all the therapists who work there to be acutely aware of public perception. If one therapist treats a client unethically, the whole business may gain a poor reputation, and the public may assume that all of the therapists act in the same way. Therapists working in businesses such as a spa where multiple therapists are employed should be very aware of what goes on around them and help educate other therapists about the importance of public perception and reputation. If another therapist sees unethical behavior, the public most likely sees it too.

One of the most common problems faced by owners of massage and bodywork businesses is the risk of poor ethical decisions made by their employees. Policies are needed on issues such as dating clients, draping, and confidentiality, but even written policies are not always followed. The policy manual should also state the conditions of and repercussions for breaking policies. For example, if a business has a policy that therapists cannot date clients, and a therapist does date a client, the repercussions could be suspension or dismissal. Policies should be clearly defined to prevent misinterpretation.

CASE STUDY

Kyle had been receiving massages at the Serenity Spa for a year and was pleased with the service. He did not really care which therapist he booked with, because so far all of his massages had been good.

This week, he had an appointment with a new therapist named Tammy. He was pleased to see that she was very attractive and about his age. During the session, she talked about herself a little, and they had good conversation. Afterwards, Kyle booked another appointment with her in the next week. Over the next few weeks, their conversations continued, and Kyle wanted to ask Tammy out. The next week, at the end of the session, Kyle asked Tammy if she would have lunch with him the next day. She accepted, and they began to see each other regularly.

A few days later Kyle mentioned to some of his buddies that he was dating his massage therapist. His buddies asked if there were other therapists there who were single and maybe open to dating. He told them the spa employed a number of therapists about their age, and his buddies asked for the telephone number of the spa. A couple of Kyle's friends called the spa and made appointments a few days later. When they booked their appointments, they asked the receptionist if their therapist was young and pretty. The receptionist answered professionally that this type of question was inappropriate. The receptionist flagged the appointments to let the therapists know that they should be cautious with these clients because of their comments. The manager of the spa too became concerned when he heard about this, and then he discovered that these clients had been referred by Kyle. After checking Kyle's records, the manager asked Tammy if she had experienced any problems with Kyle. Tammy admitted she was dating Kyle. The manager reminded Tammy of the spa's no-dating policy and said that she needed to take immediate steps to maintain her job at the spa. Tammy then spoke with Kyle and stopped seeing him in order to keep the job she loved. She had learned a valuable lesson about how her behavior could affect all the other therapists at the spa.

One therapist can affect the ethical environment of all other therapists working in the same location, as we see in the case of the therapist Tammy dating a client. How can therapists protect themselves, therefore, from possible misperceptions and inappropriate actions of others? Below are some steps therapists can take to prevent problems and protect themselves.

1. Before taking the job, check the business's policy manual and look for stated repercussions for not following policies.
2. If there is no policy manual, request that one be written.
3. Talk with a mentor.
4. Discuss with the other therapists the importance of policies and the public's perception of the business's ethics.

5. Decide how most appropriately to report therapists who do not follow policies.
6. Ask managers to enforce existing policies.

Policies work only when a business's owners and managers enforce them. All too often a company has rules but does not enforce them or uses them in an unfair way. Consistency in applying policies and procedures is crucial to the success of a business. Often people hear there are policies but know that nobody ever does anything when one is broken. Enforcing policies on a hit-or-miss basis is just as dangerous because some therapists and clients will constantly test the waters. Consistency in enforcing policies shows employees and therapists how important the policies are and what will happen if they are not followed. The same consistency in policies and enforcement also shows the public that the business cares about its policies and will enforce them. Both clients and therapists will feel safer in this environment than in one without consistency or rules. Policies that address client issues also reassure the public that the business has their well-being in mind (Fig. 11-1).

Therapists also want to know that they are being protected by the management. If a bodyworker works in a facility that does not enforce its policies, problems can occur for everyone who works there.

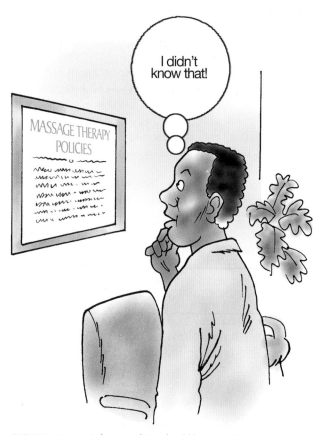

FIGURE 11-1 ■ Relevant policies should be accessible to all clients.

Asking managers to enforce policies may not make one popular, but the result of a lack of enforcement is much worse. All individual therapists should be responsible for both themselves and the environment in which they work. Being proactive about ethical concerns serves not only oneself but also the public because of the public's perception of the business. If you become the owner of a business, your policies and their enforcement should be an important focus.

REPORTING ETHICAL VIOLATIONS

When a therapist discovers unethical behavior has taken place, it is important to understand your responsibility for reporting the violation. The National Certification Board of Therapeutic Massage and Bodywork (NCBTMB) obliges therapists to report unethical behavior to the board. Other associations may also have similar obligations for their members. All therapists should know the expectations of the professional groups to which they belong and the process to be followed in these situations. Every therapist should also understand what can or will take place when a complaint is made. Read all the literature that you receive from your professional associations and groups so that you fully understand their expectations.

If you are hesitant or doubtful about reporting unethical behavior you observe, talk with a mentor to help you understand what is involved.

WORKING FOR OTHERS

When a new massage therapist enters practice, it can be scary to encounter many different issues. Many graduating students are at first unsure what type of environment they want to work in, while others have a clear picture of what they want to do. Someone entering the bodywork profession has many choices, such as spas, chiropractors' offices, medical offices including orthopedic offices, pain centers, and physical therapy facilities, resorts, outcall businesses, corporate massage (chair) settings, cruise ships, and private practice. Different facilities offer different benefits, and it is wise before choosing to become educated about the choices in your community and area. Talk with instructors, mentors, and other therapists in practice to learn more about the different expectations in different settings. The researching helps one make an educated decision about where to begin a career. Learning about a facility's policies and procedures also is an important part of the decision-making process. Check out the reputation of any facility you are interested in. Talk to friends and relatives to see what they may have heard. A Better Business Bureau in the area can tell you if any complaints have been made against a facility. State boards that oversee massage and bodywork too may provide information about specific facilities.

WORKING AS AN EMPLOYEE

Working as an employee can remove the pressure of having to manage the business side of one's own massage practice, but this does not mean that employees do not have a responsibility to work ethically. Employees are expected to follow policies and procedures developed by the owners or staff and to accept the consequences of breaking those policies and procedures. Sometimes employees feel they can do what they want once a session begins and no one is watching over them. If all employees put themselves in the place of the management, however, and took the time to understand why the rules were made, they would see that policies not only protect the business but also protect clients and the therapists. These guidelines help prevent unethical situations. For example, if a spa has a rule that clients should be draped in a certain way and a client requests no draping, the therapist can tell the client the spa's policy has to be followed. This protects the therapist and prevents cases in which a client might tell the management that a therapist acted inappropriately. With a policy that the business can refuse service to clients who behave inappropriately, if a therapist does not want to give service to a client who has made inappropriate remarks in the past, this rule helps prevent a possibly scary situation with a difficult client. Employees thereby have a sort of umbrella protection from a range of possible situations.

In addition, an employee working for others can also learn much from the experience. Other therapists and business owners who share their experience can help a new student gain tremendous insight to the bodywork business. Many students begin their careers as employees, and they can gain much by observing what works well in the bodywork industry and how different situations can be handled.

If you become an employee and later discover you are uncomfortable with the facility's ethical makeup, the best thing is to move on to a place where you can feel comfortable. The environment reflects on everyone working there, and it can take a great deal of energy to try to explain away the inappropriate actions of others. It may require some effort and research to find a place that provides the positive atmosphere you are seeking, but in turn it will provide you with a good safe place to work.

> ### Key Points
> ■ The ethical environment is a direct reflection of the owner of a business as well as everyone who works in the facility.
> ■ Policies and procedures can help address ethical situations.
> ■ Therapists should always be aware of the ethics of people who work around them.
> ■ Employees and owners should understand the repercussions of bad ethical decisions.

HOW THE ETHICS OF OTHERS AFFECT YOU

As mentioned earlier, a bodyworker's reputation can be affected by the actions of others in the facility. For example, a therapist may have the best massage technique in the city, but if this therapist is working in a place with a reputation for providing poor service, it will be difficult for even this therapist to overcome that public perception. Likewise, if a facility has a poor reputation due to past unethical situations, it will affect the reputation of all the therapists who practice there. For example, if the license of a therapist practicing in a facility was suspended for violating state rules, the public may assume that all the therapists there behave similarly. It has happened that a therapist gets into trouble and then the owners of the facility have to spend a great deal of time and money to reestablish the facility's reputation in a community. That is one reason many facilities are very careful about who they hire and why they have so many policies. It is expensive to market a business, and this effort can quickly go to waste if just one therapist makes a mistake.

Sometimes new therapists are surprised by the ethical makeup of a facility. In school you are taught to be careful with what you say and how you act with clients. When you enter the workplace, however, you will likely see some other therapists acting unprofessionally and sometimes even breaking state rules or laws. New therapists typically feel confused about what to do in such situations. If it looks like there truly could be problems, such as a rule or law being broken, talk with a mentor or former instructor. These individuals can give you guidance on what you should do.

Employees can also talk with the owner or manager of the facility about their concerns. The therapist may not be aware of everything involved in the situation, or there may be another point of view to consider. Unfortunately, some businesses continue to do things that are unethical until complaints are filed or the business is caught. Bringing an ethical issue to the manager's attention may not always lead to a solution.

If an unethical situation continues, a therapist may have to decide whether to continue to work with that business. Talk with other therapists or a mentor to clarify the situation and the alternatives. In some cases therapists leave a business and report the problem to the state board or local authorities. These are serious decisions that should not be made lightly without thought and help from others.

The actions of other therapists or managers can also raise confusing questions about what is right or wrong. Look for help to mentors, other therapists, your state board, and local ordinances as you research the problem. For example, if a therapist in a large spa with a temporary license continues to practice after the license expires, this goes against the law or ordinance. On the other hand, a therapist who keeps poor client records is not breaking the law but has poor business practices. If you discover a situation that is not illegal but you feel is unethical, view this as an opportunity to educate others about ethical practices or make the decision to seek work elsewhere. Decisions like these can take a great deal of time and energy, but it is important to deal with the situation as soon as possible.

CASE STUDY

Sandra was excited to get her first job at the Tranquility Center in her hometown. The center had been open less than a year, but it was located in one of the best shopping centers in town. Sandra felt she could build a good clientele there. Two other therapists worked in the center, and they would be sharing clients. The center seemed to have a good structure that helped everyone stay busy.

Sandra's first couple of weeks were pretty slow, however, and she was disappointed not to have more clients. One afternoon at the front desk she overheard the receptionist recommending another therapist to several people who called in for appointments. She had been told that appointments were made on a rotating basis unless the client specifically asked for a certain therapist. Later on, she asked another employee about this and learned that the therapist in question gave the receptionist an extra $5 for each appointment she booked for her. Apparently the manager did not know this was happening.

Sandra decided to talk to the owner about this. Although nothing illegal was occurring, she felt it certainly was unfair. The manager checked on this situation and discovered Sandra's allegations were true. A policy was then made that prevented any favoritism in making appointments. The receptionist learned that it was not ethical to accept special payments to book appointments.

The therapist who formerly had so many appointments became angry and threatened to ruin Sandra's business by telling clients to keep away from her. When this became known, the manager let that therapist go and then worked to restore a good relationship with the other therapists and staff.

HOW YOUR ETHICS AFFECT OTHERS

In almost all cultures, good ethical behavior is viewed in a positive, rewarding way. If you think about such people as Nelson Mandela and Mother Teresa, you realize how the caring and ethical nature of individuals like this is held in high esteem. The same is true in bodywork. The general public wants to believe that therapists behave ethically in all situations. The public wants to trust that therapists know what is right and what is wrong.

Your ethical behavior as a therapist will help you develop a reputation as someone others look to and respect. The public's respect is important because many clients come from the general public and because they also will tell others about your business.

It is also important that other professionals, including other therapists, know that you act ethically. In this competitive world, if someone says a therapist is acting unethically, this can damage that person's reputation and result in a loss of valuable business. Always think about the consequences of an action before taking it. If that action would be considered risky or unethical by someone, you should think about the possible consequences. When therapists are competing for business within a spa, for example, one might say something detrimental about another to try to get more business. This would not only affect the person talking but also affects all others who are working in the facility.

A therapist with good ethics can also teach others the positive results of acting ethically. For example, in a facility with several therapists, one therapist may be busy while others are not; this may result from not only the massage techniques used but also the ethical way in which that therapist treats clients. Clients notice even the smallest details. For example, if a therapist tells a joke that someone could consider offensive, it would be a poor choice to tell this joke to all clients. A client might be offended and tell others that he or she did not like how the therapist behaved.

Setting a good example is the best way to affect others who work around or with you. Treating clients, therapists, other employees, and the general public ethically helps others see how effective positive, ethical behavior can be.

POTENTIAL PROBLEMS

Problems sometimes occur when you work within a business. Once you recognize a problem has occurred, you need to decide whether to do nothing and let things remain the way they are or to take action. Often when a person decides to act to make a change, someone else may view the action as troublemaking or a threat to the status quo. Such decisions can be difficult to make, especially if you are the "new kid on the block." It is important to weigh a decision such as this and decide if the action will result in a positive change or just upset others. It may be better to seek other alternatives, such as seeking different employment because these decisions can be difficult. A mentor or instructor can help provide insight to such a decision-making process.

The problem that a therapist perceives could in some situations be based on information received from others, or someone else's opinion, and such information is not automatically true. Check all the facts before taking action. It would be unfortunate to take action on the basis of misinformation.

CASE STUDY

Karie had been the lead therapist at a spa for 5 years. She was responsible for training new therapists and mentoring therapists when problems arose. Therapists sometimes felt threatened by other therapists, and Karie had learned that it was always important to sort out information before taking action when a situation was brought to her.

Annie had been at the spa for only a couple of months and was disappointed that she was not very busy. Karie suggested that she provide chair massage to waiting customers and use that time to market her particular massage techniques. Later on, several of Karie's own regular clients, who had received chair massages from Annie, told Karie that Annie had said that Karie's stone massages were just a passing fad and that Annie's own new techniques would be much more relaxing for them. Karie also heard from other therapists that Annie was saying negative things to clients about their specialties.

Karie decided to talk to Annie about her conversations with clients receiving chair massage. Annie said she felt very strongly about her techniques and did not feel other types of massage were as good for clients. Karie explained that it was not ethical to try to get clients in this way. She asked Annie to put herself in the place of the other therapists and think how she would feel if they talked the same way about her techniques. Annie then understood that this was not a professional way to act; she also realized that her business had not increased by talking this way. Annie apologized to the other therapists, and they all worked with her to develop ways to describe everyone's therapies in a positive way, including hers.

If a problem occurs, never discuss it with anyone other than those involved. For example, if a client tells you that another therapist constantly talks about problems that other clients are having, it is not appropriate to tell this client that the actions violate state law or are improper. If the other therapist works at the same facility, it would be appropriate to talk with that therapist. If the therapist is not open to change or does not take the issue seriously, it may be appropriate then to talk with the facility manager. Continuing with the same example, if the therapist about whom a client complains does not work at the same facility, the seriousness of the infraction should be considered. If the client is very upset, a therapist could give the client information about options. For example, if a client is very upset about another therapist touching him or her inappropriately, the client could be told about how to file a complaint with a state board or local authorities. It is important not to become involved with another person's complaint, however, especially if you did not witness the problem.

Working with rather than against other therapists in the community is the best and most professional behavior. One should not compete for business at another therapist's expense. With some 20% of the population receiving massage therapy and bodywork, there are more than enough clients to go around. Set good ethical standards and others will see how effectively they work for you.

OWNING YOUR OWN BUSINESS

As discussed in the previous chapter, policies and procedures form a foundation and structure for a business. A business's policies should be based on how the business wants both the public and

EXERCISE 11-1

With the class divided into four groups, each group takes one of the situations below. In each discuss how the therapist should handle the situation and what, if any, action needs to be taken. Present your case to the class and discuss other suggestions from the class about other ways to handle the situation.

1. A therapist in the spa where you work continually talks negatively about other therapists who work there. She tells clients untrue things to make sure that the clients will continue to book only with her.

2. Another therapist is located close to your office. She keeps lowering her prices to compete with you. Every week her prices change, and some of your clients have begun to notice the price difference.

3. A new client states that he does not like to be draped because it makes him feel too warm. He makes a big deal about it and does not want to be draped. He tells you that he always convinces the therapist to not drape at all during his massages.

4. The owner of the facility where you work has asked you to perform a type of massage that you have never been trained for. You tell the owner that you lack the appropriate training but she tells you to go ahead and try to do some type of massage because the client will probably not know the difference.

therapists to perceive the business. Business owners who choose to not have clear-cut policies usually end up facing problems that could have been prevented. While policies are important, it is even more important to ensure that the public and clients perceive a business as having good ethical standards.

WORKING AS A SOLE PROPRIETOR

A **sole proprietor** owns and operates his or her own business. Sole proprietors generally work alone, but may work alongside other employees or independent contractors in the business. For example, three or four therapists may all work in the same office, although each works as the sole proprietor of his or her own business. The public is generally not aware of how the business is set up in an office such as this. But the public does perceive that the therapists are working together as a group. In cases such as this, it is important to know how the others act, especially when behavior involves potentially ethical issues. What one person does can easily be perceived as an action by the whole

group. Most important, any issue that arises can raise ethical questions. As noted previously, individual therapists may have their own policies about draping and dating clients, but what happens if another therapist's policies differ significantly from yours? A consensus policy that all therapists develop together and accept would help prevent possible misconceptions.

Many sole proprietors work alone, either in an office or as an out-call business. Working alone has the advantage of not being affected by the actions and ethics of other therapists. One must still be accountable to clients and any laws, rules, and regulations affecting the business. Being a professional, whether working in a group or alone, always involves being accountable for everything one does.

WORKING AS AN INDEPENDENT CONTRACTOR

Working as an **independent contractor** means that you are working independently, as your own boss, even though you may be working within a facility or business with other professionals. For example, a spa may have three massage therapists, all independent contractors, instead of three employees. This means the facility or business provides the therapists with services such as a room, supplies, and marketing in exchange for a fee or commission. Many different business structures and arrangements have developed for independent contractors in the bodywork profession. Chiropractors, spas, doctors' offices, physical therapy facilities, hospitals, and massage offices may all prefer to use independent contractors rather than employees (Fig. 11-2). Usually there are advantages for both parties.

For the facility the advantages can include:

1. Lower overhead and no hourly wages
2. No taxes or workers' compensation to be withheld from wages
3. Collective marketing done as a group, possibly dividing the costs
4. Management spends less time training and overseeing employees

For the therapist the advantages can include:

1. Setting your own schedule (within a general timeframe)
2. Being in control of your own finances
3. Control of marketing (except when participating in group marketing)
4. Being your own boss

Both parties involved in an independent contractor relationship still need to be aware of possible ethical

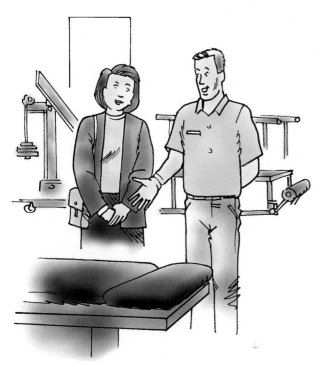

FIGURE 11-2 ■ Independent contractors may work in a physical therapy facility or many other health care settings.

issues that can arise. For example, even though a hospital allows an independent contractor to work in the facility, hospital administrators want to be sure the independent contractor will behave ethically. If the therapist were to act unethically, the public might perceive the hospital as being involved in the issue.

Therefore, it is important for both parties in an independent contractor relationship status to be acutely aware of what can happen. For example, a facility may provide a space for a therapist, but not any policies or support. Both parties should be responsible for ensuring that no unethical behavior takes place. For example, when independent contractors are working in a massage office, does this mean the owner is or is not responsible if a client is not treated ethically? In some states, the owner of such a facility has to obtain a license and is also held responsible if a problem arises.

A contract is an important component of any relationship between a business and an independent contractor. A facility in which independent contractors practice may have a standard contract for all therapists in the facility. Facilities or therapists that do not have a written contractual agreement can experience problems over even the simplest of issues. For example, a therapist may be told by an employee of the facility that he or she can book massages on Saturdays but then discover another therapist already using the room that day. If your facility does not use a standard contract,

offer to help it develop one or locate one that is agreeable to both parties. The contract should cover fees, schedule of payments, the facility's and therapists' responsibilities, shared expenses, times, booking appointments, and marketing. The contract need not be a complicated document. It can be as simple as a letter of understanding that both parties sign and date. The contract will help both parties understand issues of concern and how they are to be handled.

Independent contractors are responsible for all aspects of their business, including the environment they are practicing in. For example, if a therapist rents space in an office and later discovers that other individuals in that office are behaving unethically, what responsibilities and choices does this therapist have? Must the therapist leave and find another place to practice, or can the issues be addressed with the other individuals and resolved? Will the public's perception of the unethical business extend also to the therapist? These are all important questions that may arise when working as an independent contractor. Therapists who choose to work with this status should also be aware of the responsibilities that it involves.

Independent contractors sometimes also must face an unclear line between being independent and being an employee. In some cases, a facility does not want the responsibility of having employees yet still wants to set down the rules. The U.S. Internal Revenue Service has defined important differences between independent contractors and employees. If a therapist is working as an independent contractor, the facility cannot require set hours, fees, or uniforms for the therapist. A therapist may voluntarily agree with a facility on such guidelines, but the facility cannot make the rules for the therapist. A new massage therapist who is beginning work as an independent contractor should check IRS publications to ensure that all regulations are covered before starting to practice. Otherwise, problems may occur between the two parties. Information about "Independent Contracture of Employee" can be found in the IRS Publication 1779 "Independent Contractor or Employee" at www.ustreas.gov/.

The advantages of being your own boss, setting your own hours, and developing your own marketing strategies are very attractive to many therapists in the bodywork profession. Many therapists make this type of situation work well for them. Before entering into a contract as an independent contractor, however, first research the requirements of your state and other government agencies. Similarly, stay aware of the ethical environment that surrounds your practice.

MARKETING

Marketing one's business also involves public perceptions, which a therapist should keep in mind. The first impression potential clients form of your business may result from their perceptions of your advertising. Advertising includes business cards, newspaper or television ads, and flyers. Carefully consider what you say and what inadvertent impressions may result from any forms of advertising, because once you have used the marketing, it can be difficult to repair a misconception.

PUBLIC PERCEPTION

The goal of advertising and marketing is to get the public's attention. Observe what types of ads in a newspaper quickly get your attention, while you hardly notice others. The wording, graphics, and even placement of an ad can affect whether and how the public notices it. For example, the word "free" in an ad generally captures attention. Then the reader explores what the "free" really means in an ad. Does it require a purchase or signing a contract? "Truth in advertising" means that a business must advertise only what it truly is offering. If a business advertises something that is not available, for example, there may be legal implications, but there are certainly ethical issues involved in being truthful with potential clients.

The advertising of bodywork has raised some issues for the public. Massage and bodywork have many benefits that are frequently listed in advertising. Most commonly, advertising describes the relaxation or therapeutic benefits of massage. But some advertising has also made claims about healing properties of massage, perhaps implying that massage can heal certain illnesses. Another false claim or implication is a reduction of body weight or cellulite resulting from massage. Advertising may mislead the public to believe that they can lose weight by receiving massage. Therapists must be careful about not only what they tell clients but also what they say in any type of advertising. Many studies have confirmed the benefits of massage and

its effects on particular conditions. Providing objective information can help the public decide the likely effects of massage for them. If your advertising claims that your massage therapy has a certain effect, you should have some type of documentation to back up your claims.

Another problem is misleading advertising about the therapist's experience or training. Claiming that one is a specialist in a particular therapy carries an ethical responsibility to be proficient in the technique. Therapists have been known to add a "specialty" to their advertising after only a few hours of training. Consider whether you yourself would like to receive a "specialty" treatment from a therapist who attended only an afternoon seminar. With so many techniques and modalities available, it is the ethical responsibility of therapists to know when they are proficient and can truthfully advertise to the public about a new technique.

The language of advertising should also be scrutinized to ensure that it is not suggestive of any type of inappropriate behavior. Adjectives such as "tantalizing" or "sensual" could be misconstrued by the public to mean something other than therapeutic massage. Whenever you write an ad or promotional piece, have other people proofread it and ask them how they perceive it. A good rule is to have three or four people review the advertising to get a good sense of what the public might think.

Graphics in advertising may also evoke a response that may not be appropriate. For example, is it appropriate to show a male therapist smiling while working on a woman's bare back? This could give some people the wrong idea. A neutral facial expression might lead to a completely different perception of the picture.

Ethical advertising leads the public to believe in what a therapist does and helps give a business a good reputation. Close attention to details helps make advertising a positive marketing tool for an ethical practice.

MONEY ISSUES

Money issues often lead to legal and ethical dilemmas in all types of businesses. When a person's income or paycheck is involved, there is often a potential for misunderstanding, miscommunication, or unethical behavior. Whether a person is an employee or employer, good communication and legal documentation can help prevent such problems.

WORKING AS AN EMPLOYEE

During the interview and hiring process, much information is exchanged between a prospective employee and the hiring manager. It is easy to forget to ask questions, such as how often employees are paid or the commission for each massage. Employers may forget to mention all of the details involved in the terms of employment. In some cases an employee may later be disappointed to learn that the situation is not as good as it first seemed. For example, a spa manager may tell a therapist that the massage fee is split 50/50 with the therapist, and to a potential employee that may sound very good. But what if the manager forgot to mention that a 5% charge is deducted for expenses and overhead? Various small financial issues not detailed in the initial interview can later cause hard feelings or problems.

A therapist who is interviewing for any position should take along a list of questions about the business, hours, pay, training, and other expectations for the facility. Therapists are usually nervous during the interview process and may forget to ask questions, yet it is important to examine the facility to ensure it is the right place for them to work. All too often a new therapist starts work and later discovers problems with the pay, hours, or rules; the therapist may end up quitting and having to start the interview process all over again. Obtaining as much information as possible in the first one or two meetings helps both parties understand whether they agree on the many facets of employment. Because therapists work as both employees and independent contractors, it is important to learn the specific difference between these two types of work and to know what questions to ask.

If a business does not have clear-cut guidelines or policies about payment, commission, and fees, the therapist must clarify these issues. For example, if a business deducts certain fees for services such as laundry, is this a set fee for all therapists or does it vary based on the number of clients a therapist works on within a given pay period? Unclear situations such as this can be prevented by written documentation about all issues that relate to money. It would be unethical for a business to randomly or without notice deduct fees for services.

Ethical issues may also arise from money issues involving clients. For example, facilities have been known to add a 15% gratuity to the client's bill for services. What happens if a client feels the therapist did not do a good job and the 15% tip is not warranted? This may lead to a discussion with a manager, and a change in policy may be needed in order to keep the client happy. Some may feel that this situation should not have arisen in the first place because it should be the client's choice when and how much to tip.

Other client issues involving money may include how to deal with bad checks or credit cards. If a check is returned, does that mean the client should never receive services again? Or should such situations be handled on a case-by-case basis? A client's money issues should not be made public or available to everyone who works in a facility. For example, a receptionist who knows that a client bounced a check should not tell every hairdresser and nail tech in the spa about it. Only those who are directly involved should know, and they should be very discreet. An exception is a customer who is purposely defrauding businesses.

EMPLOYING OTHERS

Employing therapists and other support staff carries the responsibility of creating a good working atmosphere for employees and also the responsibility to assure that therapists and clients are treated fairly and ethically. The attitude of the employer sets the tone for all employees to follow.

An employer should begin with a policy and procedure manual for all employees. Policies about the payment of commission, pay periods, and fee structures should clearly outline what employees can expect. If an employee does not understand the policy or needs other arrangements made, the issue should be discussed with a manager or owner. It is unethical to talk to others about any financial disagreements with an owner or manager without first talking with that person. Clients, other therapists, and employees should not hear about these types of issues.

The previous chapter on policies and procedures described policies and procedures as living documents. The employer should write new policies or change existing policies as needed. Policies should not be written to enhance one person's career over another, but there should be flexibility for change when a policy or procedure does not provide for the clients or therapists in an appropriate way. Policies concerning finances are especially important. The policies should specify all information concerning payment amounts and schedules. Once policies and procedures are in place, it is important for owners and managers to enforce the policies fairly with staff. Not following financial policies

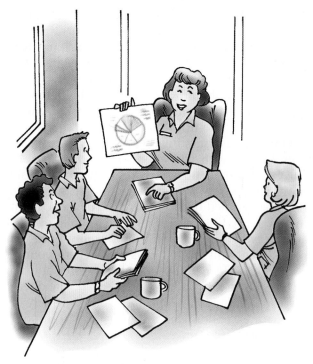

FIGURE 11-3 ■ Financial issues are frequently discussed in staff meetings.

would lead to misunderstandings and hard feelings. Showing favoritism in such policy issues is unethical and can be a major concern for those who feel they are being treated unfairly.

Many facilities have staff meetings to discuss issues, which may include policies and procedures. For example, an office with eight therapists has a meeting every month to ensure good communication and understanding about everything happening in the office. Otherwise, the eight therapists would rarely see each other due to scheduling. Staff meetings should have an open forum for everyone to discuss problems. Financial issues are frequently a topic at staff meetings (Fig. 11-3). Issues such as fee changes, commission changes, and client payments should be discussed, and all staff should be aware of any changes before they are implemented. Communicating in advance with employees about any financial issues helps prevent misperceptions that something unethical is happening.

FEE SCHEDULES

Setting fees for massage therapy and bodywork can be challenging, particularly for someone just entering the field of massage therapy. A good first step is to research what other therapists and facilities in the area charge for sessions, along with the types of services they offer. It is important to consider a therapist's training and years of experience when evaluating fees. For example, a therapist with 200 to 300 hours training in a specific modality would likely charge more than someone with only some basic training. Check with your massage school instructors, who often know current market prices. When you take continuing education courses, you can also ask the company or course instructor about reasonable fee levels. You also need to understand what your particular area accepts as a reasonable fee. For example, a destination spa may charge $105 for a Swedish massage, but in a small community $60 may be a more reasonable fee.

Setting fees for friends and family members can also be challenging. Most therapists want to offer reasonable discounts for this market, but it is important not to cut your fee to a level that you may later regret. For example, when you first begin practice you might offer your family and close friends a 1-hour massage for $30. Later on, when your practice is busy, you may find that frequent $30 massages are taking up part of your schedule and displacing clients who pay your normal rate of $65. It is important to determine reasonable and acceptable fees for friends and family without becoming resentful.

Clients often tell therapists that they do not have the money for regular massage sessions. They may ask for a discount. A potential solution is to set up a sliding scale. A sliding scale determines the fee based on a client's income. For example, a client who makes $25,000 a year may pay $40 for a massage, while a client who makes $40,000 may pay your normal rate of $60. A sliding scale should be used consistently with all your clients, however. This is a way of providing fair and equitable care for all your clients and potential clients.

TIPS AND TAXES

All employees and business owners have a personal responsibility to know and understand all tax laws and rules that apply to them. Unfortunately, some individuals do not follow local, state, or federal tax rules. Violations of these laws can cause many problems including penalties and interest payments due as well as potential criminal actions. Too many people think they can avoid paying tax when they accept cash for services. Tips and even bartered services, however, are considered taxable income. The service industry is well known for people accepting cash and not reporting it to the government or paying taxes on this income. Anyone going into a service business should talk with an accountant to learn what rules apply and to set up a financial plan. For example, independent contractors pay their own taxes. An accountant can set up a quarterly payment plan to avoid a big tax bill at the end of the year. Accountants can also explain the many tax deductions available to those who own their own business.

GIFT CERTIFICATES

Gift certificates will be an important part of your business as a massage therapist. During several holidays throughout the year, such as Valentine's Day and Mother's Day, therapists can make substantial income by selling gift certificates.

Several things need to be considered when offering gift certificates. First, do any state laws apply to the selling of gift certificates? In some states, it is illegal to put an expiration date on a gift certificate. Laws protect the public from businesses that sell gift certificates but do not honor them. Even if your state does allow an expiration date, how would people feel if they cannot redeem a gift certificate that has expired? A therapist might be tempted to consider this an easy way to earn income because a certain percentage of gift certificates are never redeemed or are redeemed after the expiration date. An ethical way to view the redemption of a gift certificate is money has been received and that a client who receives quality services will tell others about the business. Everyone who receives a gift certificate is a potential new client and may tell others about your business. Some therapists keep track of gift certificate purchases, and when one is not redeemed after a reasonable time, they call the purchaser and offer to provide the services that were purchased. This is an ethical goodwill gesture to clients and potential clients. Many businesses use gift certificates as an effective part of their marketing plan.

Therapists are often asked to donate gift certificates to fundraisers or to new clients to market their business. For example, someone in your community who is known for talking with many people about town is a good candidate to receive a massage gift certificate. After all, such a person is likely to tell everyone how good your massages are. Find two or three of these individuals and your marketing expenses can dramatically drop.

Key Points
■ Good communication and legal documentation can help prevent problems.
■ It is important for a prospective employee to ask questions regarding all money issues.
■ Expectations should be written in the form of policies and procedures.

SUMMARY

Business ethics involves both personal ethics and the ethics of others in the workplace. It is important to be aware of the behavior and attitude of others in your workplace, as their behavior reflects on everyone there. Policies can set the tone, but employers should pay close attention to compliance for the safety and well-being of both clients and therapists. If unethical behavior is allowed to happen or is ignored, the business could develop a poor reputation with the public. Good ethical behavior helps to build a business's reputation in a profession where ethics are very important.

12

CONFLICT RESOLUTION

- Conflicts that occur between therapists and clients, other therapists, employers, and other health care professionals
- Conflicts that occur when needs change
- Resolving conflicts step by step

KEY TERMS

Conflict: a condition that occurs when two or more people have different attitudes or ideas about how something should be done or when a person has to choose between two inconsistent actions

Resolution: a solution found or formulated to end a conflict

Conflicts and differences of opinion are inevitable when working with or providing services to others. The expectations of others involved in a practice are not always the same. Clients, other therapists, employers, and employees frequently change their expectations, and a therapist needs to be open and flexible enough to allow changes to happen. Clients can change their expectations from session to session or even within a session. Growth involves change, and working toward a positive **resolution** for conflicts is an important step for those in any service industry. Conflicts can happen when there is a difference of opinion between two parties on an ethical issue. The resolution of a conflict can help a business be more productive and in some cases helps ensure that the public is being treated ethically. This chapter explains areas where conflict can happen and why, and describes steps that can be taken to help resolve conflicts.

WHY CONFLICTS HAPPEN

Almost everyone resolves conflicts on a daily basis in their personal and business lives. Because many conflicts are easily resolved, they may not involve much thought or stress. For example, when arriving at a four-way-stop intersection, three drivers may be unsure who arrived first, and usually for a few moments everyone is trying to decide who goes next. Eventually someone moves first and then everyone moves along. It would be great if all conflicts were this easily handled, but in many cases the conflict takes considerable time and effort to resolve.

Conflicts can also occur when a difference of opinion occurs regarding an ethical issue. For example, one therapist in a business may believe that it is unethical to share a client's records with another therapist, while others may not see an ethical dilemma here. Another example arises when a client wants to socialize with a therapist. There are often many different opinions about this situation.

People often justify their actions when explaining why they did something. If a therapist is questioned about an action, it may mean that another party believes the action was not the most effective or appropriate. Certain actions have ethical implications. Because there are a variety of opinions about most ethical issues, therapists must consider what they are willing to take ownership of in their own code of ethics or have agreed to follow in a group or professional association.

A seminar was held on ethics with more than 50 therapists attending. The age and experience of the therapists varied widely and represented a good cross section of therapists in the bodywork profession. There were teachers, new graduates, and therapists who had been in the field for many years.

One of the graduates asked a good question during the seminar: "Is it okay to accept social invitations from your clients?" She explained that one of her clients frequently offered her tickets to a sporting event. She did not feel right accepting them, but other therapists in her spa said that she should accept them. She did not feel good about the offers, and the client seemed a little too friendly.

This question led to a great deal of discussion and variety of opinions. Several therapists said it was okay to accept social invitations, while others believed it was clearly a boundary issue. An intense debate followed. Finally, near the end after a number of people expressed some very strong opinions on the matter, an older experienced therapist stood up and said, "If you feel strongly enough about anything, you can easily justify it in your own mind. What is important to note is that if you are having to justify your behavior to several people, maybe you should take a second look at that behavior."

Often people will perceive what they want about another's actions or behavior. Many therapists go through their entire careers without ever being questioned about their behavior or actions. Obviously they are very aware of the impressions they give others and choose not to behave in any way that would lead to ethical questions.

Justifying and explaining one's behavior may be necessary in certain professions and fields of work. But therapists who are frequently questioned about their actions should take a close look at what they are doing and adjust their behavior accordingly.

UNCLEAR EXPECTATIONS

Many times a conflict arises when one or both parties have unclear expectations regarding the other party. For example, in a practice with several therapists, one therapist may expect the other therapists to always be neat and clean up after themselves after each day's work. Although this may sound like common sense to many, some therapists prefer instead to clean up before they start in the morning.

Unclear expectations can arise when a person's own guidelines and habits are not the same as those of others around them. Often a person will assume that others should have the same work habits and guidelines, but the variety of backgrounds and situations in which people are raised lead to a variety of work habits and behaviors. Previous chapters discussed policy and procedures, which can help give individuals guidelines to follow. Unfortunately, even the best policies and procedures sometimes still involve individual interpretation, and the expectations of one person may be very different from another's. An owner of a facility may assume, for example, that all the therapists will follow the same ethical guidelines, only to be surprised when a complaint is filed against a therapist charging unethical behavior. Policies and procedures can help in many ways but often are still somewhat open to interpretation.

Expectations frequently change, and it can be frustrating to have conflicts develop even when a policy has been in place for a considerable period of time. Sometimes there are no policies for a given situation because a problem has never occurred with it in the past, allowing a conflict to suddenly develop.

Lawrence has run an office with three other therapists in a great location for the last 3 years. Their business was in the heart of a successful business district, and their advertising budget was low because they had good exposure to the public. In the past, Lawrence and the other therapists had verbally agreed to an advertising budget. Now Lawrence received word that the major street where they were located was being re-routed and their street in the future would have only walking traffic. Lawrence realized that this would be a problem because direct parking by the building would no longer be available and the office sign would be hard to see.

Lawrence decided that they were going to have to spend a lot more money on an advertising budget to keep up the business. Lawrence expected the other therapists to agree with what he had decided.

During a meeting with the therapists, Lawrence announced the new budget and what he expected each of them to contribute. His therapists were independent contractors who rented space from him. One of the therapists thought the plan was good, but the other two disagreed with his new budget. Lawrence had calculated the budget and divided it four ways for all to share equally in the expenses. Since the therapists were independent contractors, however, he could not require them to pay the new expenses. Lawrence had just expected them to want to advertise and spend the money to help maintain their businesses.

Several business and ethical dilemmas are evident here. If the other therapists signed a rental/lease agreement, Lawrence may have the option to raise the rent to cover the new expenses. Is it ethical for Lawrence to raise the rent for this type of situation, or should he allow them to be released from their lease? If the therapists do not like what is happening, is it ethical for them to vacate suddenly and leave Lawrence in the lurch for these expenses?

All the parties entered into their original agreement with certain expectations, but due to unforeseen circumstances, the expectations changed. When a situation occurs that may cause conflict, resolution and compromise should be sought.

Unclear expectations can often be avoided by careful planning and communication. It is not a good idea to assume that other therapists or your employer will know your expectations unless they are clearly outlined and stated.

Clients can also have unclear expectations about the therapy they are going to receive and the therapeutic relationship. For example, a client may assume that the therapeutic relationship means that a therapist can treat any kind of ailment. Massage therapists should not work on many conditions, however, but should explain to clients why their condition does not warrant bodywork. A recent neck trauma such as whiplash, for example, often requires medical assessment before bodywork is performed. It is unethical and beyond the scope of practice for a bodyworker to work on clients who could potentially be harmed or whose conditions contraindicate massage. Explaining the scope of massage therapy can help a client understand that a massage therapist or bodyworker has parameters they must practice within. Referring the client appropriately would be the ethical thing to do.

Clients can also have expectations for the therapy session itself. A client may expect the therapist to make them 100% better in just one session. Experienced therapists know to educate their clients about the long-term process of working on a chronic or established condition. Years of problems and pain cannot magically disappear in a 1-hour session. Conditions such as arthritis, injuries, and long-term overuse are frequent maladies that clients suffer. Clients often tell the therapist that they want to get rid of the pain in their shoulder, for example. Therapists can educate clients about how long it took the condition to develop and explain that it may take a series of sessions to make a long-term improvement. Clients may also expect a therapist to be an expert in other matters that

pertain to health. Often clients ask a therapist to diagnose what is wrong with them. Because therapists are trained in pathologies, clients expect a therapist to know what is wrong with them. Clients often list all types of symptoms and then ask the therapist what is wrong with them. Therapists are trained in pathologies to help them recognize when it is not appropriate to work on a person or area to prevent harming a client. Diagnosing is beyond the scope of practice for a bodyworker; yet clients frequently ask a therapist what is wrong with them. Therapists should be careful how they word their answers to such questions. In cases such as these, referring the client to another health care professional for a diagnosis is the proper thing to do. Clients may also expect a therapist to have knowledge about medications and supplements. Again, it is beyond the scope of practice for a bodyworker to advise a client to take or not take medications and supplements (Fig. 12-1). Even a client who simply asks if taking a certain vitamin will help with a condition is asking the therapist to answer beyond a therapist's scope of practice. Referring such clients to their physician or another health care professional is appropriate because nutrition and medications are beyond the scope of practice for bodyworkers.

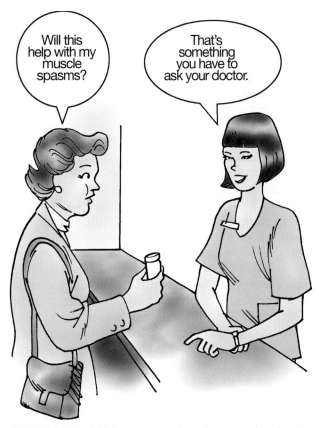

FIGURE 12-1 ■ Advising clients about supplements and medications is outside the scope of practice of massage therapy.

Key Points

- Unclear expectations can cause conflict.
- Planning and communication can help avoid conflict.
- Expectations should be stated or expressed by all parties involved.

CROSSING BOUNDARIES

Therapists should be knowledgeable of the boundaries of their profession. Laws, rules, regulations, and the codes of ethics of professional associations or groups must be followed. Problems can arise when an individual either is not aware of such boundaries or chooses not to accept them. For example, a therapist may not be aware of a state rule requiring a client to give informed consent to receive bodywork. Informed consent, as discussed previously, means that a client is given information about a treatment prior to the treatment and consents to it after receiving all pertinent information. If a therapist does not tell a client that a certain technique may cause side effects, for example, a client may become upset when the side effects happen. Ignorance of the law or rules is not an acceptable defense. It is the responsibility of all therapists to know what is required of them by rules and laws. Knowing the expectations can prevent potential conflicts. Otherwise, a client or another therapist might report the therapist for a rule violation, and a state board may send an inspector or letter concerning the violation.

A therapist who deliberately chooses to cross legal or ethical boundaries certainly raises an ethical issue. The National Certification Board of Therapeutic Massage and Bodywork has increased the required number of continuing education hours in ethics from 2 to 6 hours. Many other professional organizations also now require more hours in ethics as a consequence of the increasing number of violations. Ethical violations can result in a report sent to a state agency or a professional organization. In some cases, violations involve a therapist not following a rule, but in other cases a conflict occurs between a therapist and a client. For example, what happens if a client feels that a therapist did not provide full information regarding a treatment? Is the client doing the right thing to file a complaint? Or should this situation be resolved at the client–therapist level? Conflicts can develop between a client and a therapist when expectations are not clearly defined between them or when information is not provided that would help both parties know what to expect or to provide. For example, if a client chooses not to tell a therapist about a certain medical condition and the bodywork makes the client's condition worse as a result, who should be held accountable?

Often violations result from boundaries being crossed. Although some boundaries may be crossed inadvertently, it is the responsibility of therapists to know what the legal and ethical boundaries are and to explain them to their clients. Clients can innocently ask that something be done that would require a therapist to cross boundaries, such as diagnosing. But what if the therapist gives a client an opinion concerning what is wrong with the client? This could lead to some serious problems and consequences for both the client and the therapist.

Clients look to a therapist as being educated in many areas concerning their health and well-being. Because bodyworkers understand the human body, it is natural that some clients might assume that a therapist can help them with their health problems. Therapists have to be careful not to overstep the boundaries of their scope of practice. If a therapist tells clients that they may have a certain medical condition, this is not only a scope of practice issue but an ethical issue as well. For example, if these clients tell their doctor that their massage therapist told them they have a skin cancer, the doctor would question the ethics of that therapist. Conflicts could easily develop between different health care providers, with the client potentially caught in the middle.

CASE STUDY

Addison had begun working on a client who had several health issues. During her sessions, the client would consistently talk about her health problems in the last week and was frustrated with not feeling very well. Addison heard her mention a number of symptoms that Addison's own sister had recently experienced before being diagnosed with diabetes. Then the client asked her if she had heard of anything that could help her with her condition and symptoms. Without thinking, Addison said that it sounded like she may have diabetes, because she had the same symptoms her sister had. The client got very upset and asked Addison what to do. Addison recommended that she see her health care provider. During a session a few weeks later, the client told Addison that she had been tested for diabetes and that the test was negative, but she had been diagnosed with a hormone problem that required medication.

Although Addison was correct in referring the client, she would have been wiser not to mention diabetes but to suggest only that the symptoms she was experiencing could be clarified by a qualified health care provider.

Boundaries help to protect clients and therapists. When a therapist or client crosses over a boundary, the potential is set for conflicts to happen. For example, if a client later learns that a therapist was supposed to have all clients fill out a health history form but did not do so, a conflict may arise. The therapist may not accurately understand the client's condition and might perform a therapy that could harm the client. This client may file a complaint or simply not return as a client. Addressing issues such as these helps prevent the conflict and the potential for clients not being happy with their therapist.

> ### Key Points
>
> ■ Therapists should know the boundaries of their profession.
> ■ Conflicts and ethical dilemmas often involve boundary issues.
> ■ Boundaries protect both clients and therapists.

POOR COMMUNICATION

Effective communication between a therapist and clients, other therapists, and an employer is important to help prevent conflicts. Expectations and boundaries can be verbalized or written to help prevent anyone from having incorrect expectations.

Written communication includes statements, rules, or policies presented to a client and signed by the client before treatment is rendered. Intake forms often state what a therapist is able and not able to do. The forms may state that a therapist does not diagnose or perform spinal manipulations, for example, to make it clear to clients that this is beyond the massage therapy scope of practice. Clients may still ask for these things, but a written and signed form helps make this policy clearer for clients and helps prevent a conflict with a client asking for something that should not be done.

Verbal communication happens continuously in a therapeutic relationship. After the initial intake interview, a therapist should seek feedback often from the client. A client's expectations cannot be met if the therapist does not have a clear picture of them. For example, if a client regularly has a relaxation massage, the therapist might naturally assume that their next session would be for relaxation. But what if the client has hurt his or her shoulder and wants the therapist's help to reduce the pain and lack of movement in that shoulder? Talking with the client would clarify that goal. You might assume that clients will always tell you what they want or expect, but unfortunately many do

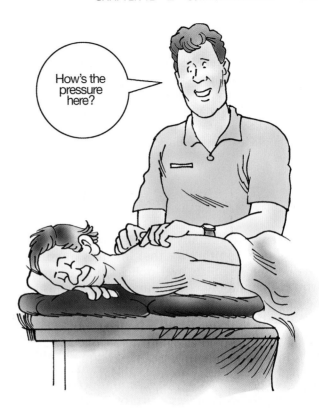

FIGURE 12-2 ■ Seek feedback often from the client during a session.

not feel comfortable talking to a therapist about their needs. For example, clients commonly complain to other people about how much pressure a therapist applies—but do not say anything to the massage therapist. Too often such a client says very little but does not return for another appointment and may never want to receive a massage again. Again, simply asking clients how they feel and if the pressure is comfortable helps prevent such problems (Fig. 12-2).

When a client does communicate a need, such as for less pressure, therapists should listen and follow what the client is telling them. If the therapist tries to convince a client that the client needs something else, a potential for conflict rises. For example, if the client tells the therapist that the pressure being used hurts, it is inappropriate for the therapist to answer that the client really needs this type of pressure. **When clients communicate their needs, it is important for the therapist to listen carefully.** If a client is not communicating, it is important for the therapist to ask for feedback to ensure the client's needs are being met.

Good communication involves constantly checking in with clients, fellow therapists, and employers to help prevent conflicts from developing. When a conflict does occur, using the process described later in this chapter helps to resolve issues.

> *Key Points*
> - Communication between the client and therapist can help prevent conflicts.
> - A therapist should focus on both verbal and nonverbal communication from a client.
> - If a client does not communicate, the therapist should ask for feedback.

TYPES OF CONFLICTS

Conflict is likely in any type of business that provides service to others or that involves more than one person. Conflicts over policies, procedures, or working conditions are common and can usually be easily resolved. Conflicts that occur over objective questions and issues are generally more easily resolved that those involving subjective feelings and beliefs. Ethical principles, although obvious at times, often involve subjective issues that can lead to conflicts if not addressed. Communicating when problems arise is a key part of resolution, but unfortunately effective communication does not always occur.

CONFLICTS WITH CLIENTS

Conflicts between a therapist and client usually result from unclear expectations by one or both of the parties. When clients book an appointment for bodywork, they generally have a certain expectation, often the same as when they book an appointment with a doctor. They usually expect the doctor to tell them what is wrong and prescribe a treatment or medication to make them better. The same is true of people who book a bodywork session. They may expect pain relief or simple relaxation from stress.

It is important for a therapist to try to learn the client's expectations through verbal and physical communication. In the initial intake process, ideally the client form requests clients to write their goals for the session. The therapist should then discuss this with the client and come to an agreement about what the client wants from the session. A client with a neck or shoulder injury may expect a therapist to fix this condition in one session. The client should be educated about the work to be performed along with the outcomes before a session begins. A client could be very disappointed with the session if told at the end of a session that a session can only accomplish so much and that the client needs to return for a long series of sessions. Clients may think that this is just a way to

keep them coming back. Telling a client about how long it took a condition to develop and how massage works best when done slowly and not aggressively will help the client understand and heal more effectively.

Clients' needs frequently change, and it is important for a therapist to address these before each session begins. Asking clients about their goals before each session helps the therapist know what they expect. Restating their goals helps to clarify the need and also allows the therapist to explain what type of work they may be doing that day. Entering the session with clear goals and expectations helps both the client and therapist know what to do and expect (Fig. 12-3).

Conflicts arise when the expectations are not clearly defined or not discussed at all. Unfortunately, a client who is not happy with a session may simply just go away and not return for future sessions. The client may not express his or her dissatisfaction to the therapist or receptionist. For example, if a client expects a deep tissue massage but receives a Swedish massage, what might the client do? Talking to the manager is a possible first step, and that may lead to a good solution. But what if the therapist feels the client did receive a deep tissue massage? Many therapists work directly with clients without others involved who can help resolve a conflict, and if a

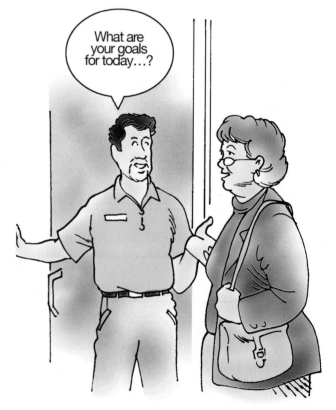

FIGURE 12-3 ■ Starting every session with clear goals helps both the client and therapist know what to do and expect.

client is unhappy with the work, what can be done? The therapist may provide another session or refer the client to another therapist to resolve the problem.

Obtaining feedback from a client during and after a session helps the therapist address the client's needs and expectations. During the session the therapist should check in with the client about pressure and comfort three or four times. Each time a different area of the body is being worked, a therapist should simply ask if the pressure is okay. Signs of discomfort such as a client tightening up or pulling away are indications that something needs to be changed or addressed. Make sure the client is warm enough, because a client who has been cold during the entire session is not going to feel relaxed at the end.

After a session, check in with the client again to ask how he or she feels and if there are any questions about the session or the expected outcomes. This is a good time to review what the client's expectations were for the session and talk about future sessions when applicable. Communicating with the client after the session is over helps the therapist gain valuable feedback and can help plan future sessions if the client is returning.

If a conflict does arise, such as clients feeling like their needs were not met or they did not receive the type of therapy they asked for, the conflict should be resolved as quickly as possible. Ask the client what expectations were not met and what solution the client would be happy with. This may mean that the client does not pay for a session or next time asks for another therapist. Unfortunately, a therapist may not always be a perfect match for every client. For example, a client who likes really deep work will not be satisfied with a therapist who only does light work. Therefore, the therapist should talk with the potential client when the appointment is booked and ask the client what type of work he or she is seeking. In facilities where a receptionist books appointments, the problem is more likely to happen if the receptionist is not educated about the types of treatments each therapist performs. Educating staff is important in such a facility.

Resolving the conflict helps show clients that their well-being is important. Refer the client to another therapist who will perform the type of work the client is looking for, and the client will respect you for doing so. Ethics involves putting a client's well-being foremost. Massage therapy is a service industry and therapists should strive to meet clients' needs. If a therapist is simply just doing the job and has no concern for the client's expectations and outcomes, satisfactory services are not being provided. Most ethical codes, therefore, address the well-being of clients.

CASE STUDY

Brett booked an appointment at the Blue Nile Day Spa for a deep tissue massage. Brett had begun jogging a few months previously and found that a deep tissue massage once a month really helped him feel better. He asked the receptionist about the deep tissue massage and asked for a therapist who could do this deep work. She told him that all five therapists did deep tissue work.

Brett had the massage on Saturday and was surprised when he was escorted to the room without first even meeting his therapist. Olivia, the therapist, entered the room and simply asked him how he was doing and proceeded to work. Brett felt the work he was receiving was too light and several times asked Olivia to work deeper. Each time she would work slightly harder, but never to the pressure that he expected from a deep tissue massage. When the session was over, Olivia left the room without saying much at all.

When Brett paid for his session, the receptionist asked if everything went well. Brett told her that he felt he had received a Swedish massage and not deep tissue work. The receptionist asked Olivia about this, and she admitted she had not looked at the appointment book before beginning and had indeed performed a relaxation massage. The manager overheard this and offered Brett a free session the next time he came in.

Situations like these can be avoided when the expectations of both parties are discussed prior to the massage rather than assumed.

CONFLICTS WITH OTHER THERAPISTS

Practices involving more than one person can have, and usually do have, many differing perspectives and ethical standards. Group practices also have the potential for a variety of conflicts because of different beliefs in policies and procedures, skills, techniques, advertising, dress, fees, and general office environment. Groups often face the challenge of working through various conflicts that can occur. Successful group practices often have regular office meetings to discuss issues before they have a chance to get out of hand. Groups such as these usually have developed ways to resolve conflicts to keep the focus on the clients and not the issues in the office.

Conflicts in a group setting also include conflicts between therapists. When they occur, it is best to try to resolve the issue between these two people and not involve other staff who may take sides and allow the problem to grow. People often seek out the advice of others, but this may allow a simple problem to grow into something larger. For example, if two therapists share a room and there is a problem with scheduling or cleaning the room, this problem should be resolved between the two parties and not the rest of the staff. If a problem arises that does involve the entire staff, meeting together would be the best approach to find a resolution. For example, if a landlord plans to increase maintenance fees in a way that affects everyone in the office, a meeting should be called to discuss the change. Otherwise, business and ethical conflicts can divert much productive energy away from the therapeutic aspect of a bodywork business.

CASE STUDY

Massage Connection opened with five therapists on staff. Careful planning by the five therapists made them all feel this would be a great place to work. Several months after opening, four of the therapists had pretty full schedules. The other therapist was still struggling to get clients. This therapist began to gossip about the other therapists. Some of the things she said got back to the other therapists in the practice. Initially, they ignored the talk, but eventually it got out of hand. Clients frequently told them things they had heard, even that some sexual improprieties had occurred in cross-gender massages. The four therapists decided to try to resolve the issue. Meeting with the therapist who was gossiping, they learned that she felt like something like this must be going on because they were getting clients and she was not. The four therapists explained that they were not doing these things and that her gossip was hurting everyone, including herself. They explained that her own unethical actions, such as gossiping, were hurting her own practice. After all, how can a client trust a therapist who is constantly gossiping about everyone else? The four therapists felt strongly that if this therapist did not stop behaving this way, they would have to ask her to leave the practice. They also offered to mentor her in ways to improve her own skills to help build a successful practice. She agreed and, a year later, was busy with her practice.

Group dynamics play an important role in conflicts and resolution. Carefully selecting other therapists with whom to practice can help prevent conflicts from occurring.

CASE STUDY

Massage Associates had six therapists who shared space in an office. During the last 5 years, several therapists had come and gone. Four of the six therapists had been together since the beginning, and they found that it was important for all four to agree on any new therapists who would join their office. They had seen that hasty decisions had brought about problems involving scheduling, advertising, and the atmosphere of the office. The last therapist who left had wanted to change the entire structure of the office and had constantly talked with all of the therapists privately to get her way. That eventually led to the four therapists asking her to leave the office because it took too much time and energy to deal with her.

The four therapists then decided to individually interview any potential therapist who wanted to practice in their facility. They felt it was important for everyone to feel comfortable with any therapist who wanted to join their office. This allowed four different perspectives and gave each individual a say in the makeup of their office.

Group practices can present challenges different from those in an employer/employee situation. When a conflict occurs in an employer/employee facility, often the employer has the final say in what happens. In a group practice, a community decision is often needed. This may involve more effort because all parties' opinions should be taken into consideration and a compromise may be needed.

A therapist who is considering joining a group situation should talk with everyone involved. It requires a large investment of time, money, and energy to start a practice, either with a group or individually. Researching the practice location and getting to know everyone there helps prevent problems later. Meeting with the staff and getting a general sense of the office's atmosphere, guidelines, and expectations for everyone helps lead to an informed decision. How busy the practice is should not be the only factor for choosing a practice.

CASE STUDY

Tia had recently relocated to Chicago from Dallas when her husband's company transferred him. She had practiced in a chiropractic office in Dallas, but had been exploring the thought of joining in a group practice. She felt out of touch with her profession and thought this might be a way to network more effectively. She saw several promising ads in the newspaper and set up appointments to meet with several groups.

Her first appointment left her discouraged and disappointed. The therapist who acted as office manager quickly showed her the office and rooms, told her the rent, and basically said everyone was on their own. When Tia tried to ask her questions about office policies and guidelines, the therapist told her that they all did their own thing.

Tia had a better experience at the second location. One of the therapists took the time to give her a tour, showed her the office policy manual, and explained a great deal about the practice. She introduced her to several of the therapists who were between sessions and told Tia that she would need to meet with all of the therapists in the office. They would discuss the fit and let her know how they felt about her joining their office. The therapist explained that this was to help avoid conflicts. She also suggested that Tia receive a massage from several of the therapists in the office to get to know what the office felt like and what type of work everyone did. The entire staff liked to be able to offer a variety of different types of therapies to help attract more clients.

Tia booked several sessions over the following weeks and found that she really liked the atmosphere and professional image of the office. She met with each of the staff, and even though it took over a month to go through the process, Tia felt the effort was worth it. She opened her practice in the location a few weeks later and found that her practice grew quickly. She attributed her success to doing research and finding the right fit with the other therapists at the facility. She easily fit into the area, and the networking opportunities were great.

CONFLICTS WITH EMPLOYERS

When one works as an employee, the ethical standards of the employer are generally the accepted standard that all employees are expected to follow. Problems are more common in workplaces when the employer does not have set standards or the standards are too tight or too loose. For example, some therapists might feel a spa's guidelines are too restrictive if they cannot work on the gluteal area. Or if a spa has no guidelines when it comes to draping, does that mean that anything goes? Do therapists look then to state laws and rules for their standards? What if the state does not have these guidelines? What will make the clients feel safe and comfortable? In such situations bodyworkers and therapists frequently have questions about what to do. Employers who want to assure the safety and comfort of their clients should take the time to

address these issues that a client and therapist could face. If not, clients may inadvertently or purposely test a therapist to see what will happen. Employers should support the therapists who work for them to ensure that when they are alone with a client in a therapy room, there is little room for anything inappropriate to happen.

CASE STUDY

Howard was pleased to be able to take his first vacation from Massage-On-The-Go in 3 years. He had worked hard to build up a good reputation for his business and had worked consistently with local authorities to help provide a safe environment for his therapists to go on out-calls. He worked with each therapist to assure that the services for the clients were reputable.

While out of town, he got a call that one of his therapists had been arrested for illicit behavior. He was shocked because he had done everything he could to hire people he knew he could trust. The male therapist had a complaint filed against him by a woman's husband. The husband had come home while his wife was receiving a massage and was upset that the therapist was working on his wife's gluteal area. The therapist had carefully draped the client and had asked her if she felt comfortable. The husband felt it was not appropriate, however, and ordered the therapist to leave and then called the police. Howard wanted to help the therapist with this problem, and he hired a lawyer to defend the therapist. Although the therapist had followed state guidelines and local regulations, the client's husband felt he had cause to file a complaint. Later in court, the therapist was proved innocent, but it was a valuable lesson for everyone to recognize that even when rules and regulations are followed, others often have different perceptions of ethical behavior. In this case, the employer supported and worked with the therapist to resolve the conflict that could affect them both.

When working for another person, it is important to understand that person's expectations. Putting expectations in writing can help all parties involved know what is and is not tolerated. Because ethics can be very subjective, it is important to be specific in any areas that might be unclear. Employers should be open to listen to the needs and concerns of their employees as well as to address clients' well-being (Fig. 12-4).

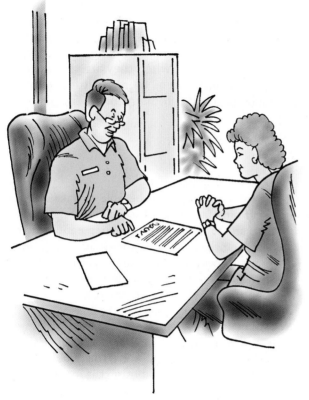

FIGURE 12-4 ■ An employer's expectations should be based on ethical behavior and be clarified in written policies.

CONFLICTS WITH OTHER HEALTH CARE PROFESSIONALS

It is becoming increasingly common for therapists to work with a variety of other health care providers in the community. As the need for massage grows, more health care providers use massage therapists and bodyworkers to help address many health issues for their clients and patients. Some use bodywork as an adjunct therapy to enhance the effects of what they are doing, while others refer a client or patient specifically for a massage for a particular condition. Many therapists actively seek out referrals from other health care providers. For example, a neuromuscular therapist may seek referrals from an orthopedic specialist because this type of therapy is known to help many conditions treated by this medical specialty.

When a massage therapist develops a relationship with other health care providers, it is important for both parties to know the other party's expectations (Box 12-1). For example, a doctor may expect the therapist to work on a patient for six sessions and only six. The therapist may expect to work on the patient until the patient feels better. This could easily lead to a conflict between the two parties, and referrals may stop. Simple ground rules can be established between the two referring parties to prevent conflict and maintain a good working relationship to benefit patients or clients.

■ **Know the expectations.** Establish ground rules both parties agree to. This may include what types of therapy, timeframes, billing, costs, and communication.
■ **Put the client/patient first.** The client's well-being should always be in the forefront. If a therapist does not agree with a diagnosis or treatment, it should be discussed with the other health care provider, not the patient.
■ **Communication.** Good communication between the two providers can build a strong professional relationship and provide good service to patients/clients.

Conflicts can and will happen between clients and their therapists, between two therapists, between employers and employees, and with other health care providers. Often these conflicts involve ethical issues. Communicating with and understanding the expectations of all parties helps prevent conflicts from occurring. When conflicts do occur, steps should be taken as quickly as possible to resolve the conflict. The complexity of ethical issues, along with their importance, makes careful resolution necessary.

Key Points

■ It is important to know both parties' expectations.
■ Expectations can frequently change.
■ Group dynamics play an important role in conflicts and resolution.
■ Policies and procedures can help prevent conflicts.
■ Conflicts between a therapist and client can be prevented with good communication.

STEPS FOR CONFLICT RESOLUTION

Conflicts can happen in any profession, and professionals generally agree that resolution is needed if the business is to succeed and grow. For example, a company that frequently receives complaints about its services could quickly go out of business if it did not act to resolve the complaints. The time and energy that conflict takes away from a business can be overwhelming.

Box 12-2 lists steps that can be taken to help resolve conflict. These steps can be used to resolve all types of conflicts between massage therapists and clients, other therapists, employers, and other health care professionals. Follow through the steps in the order listed to reach a positive outcome.

BOX 12-2	*Steps for Conflict Resolution*

1. Identify the person(s) involved.
2. Identify the problem(s).
3. Research the facts.
4. Consider possible solutions and outcomes.
5. Discuss solutions with all parties involved.
6. Compromise and resolve.

IDENTIFY THE PERSON(S) INVOLVED

Often a conflict is between just two people, but other people may get involved in the problem or process. Problems can easily get out of hand as more people get involved. A variety of opinions may be offered, and some people may even enjoy watching the chaos that may result from conflict. It is best to quickly identify the key people involved in the conflict. Look back to the beginning of the conflict and identify the people who were taking part. Eliminate anyone else from the discussion except for the key figures in the problem. Otherwise, many people often want to get involved in the drama of a situation and offer their opinion about it.

IDENTIFY THE PROBLEM(S)

When a conflict arises it is important to take the time to write down what the problem is. Often a conflict involves strong emotions, such as frustration or anger. Being objective can be challenging when emotions are involved. Writing down a problem can help one be more objective and less emotional. Try to stay objective and list just the facts of the conflict. As well, try to see the situation from the other person's perspective. Think about how they may feel about the actions taken by other parties involved.

RESEARCH THE FACTS

It is important to put emotions aside and look strictly at the facts. For example, if your office is having scheduling conflicts, it is important to determine who is involved and look at the appointment book and time cards to help determine the facts of the scheduling problem. Write down just the facts of the situation. When researching the facts, keep opinions—both your own and others—out of this process.

CONSIDER POSSIBLE SOLUTIONS AND OUTCOMES

For every problem there is usually more than one possible solution. It is human nature, however, to see only one answer to a problem and then focus on that. But when you are dealing with one or more other people, the range of resolutions can be as different as night and day. Have all the parties involved write down their possible solutions to the problem. Try to explore all possible options. For example, for the scheduling conflict, the solution may be something as simple as a schedule readjustment. But it could also require a major overhaul of the entire staff's schedule to repair the situation. Try to find as many solutions to the problem as you can, and then write down the likely outcome from each. It is obvious that the conflict should be resolved, but it is important to determine how the different outcomes will affect other parties.

This may be a good time to ask for assistance from a mentor. Ask the mentor to read what you have written to this point, and ask for additional input and possible solutions. A mentor who has worked in the bodywork field may have valuable insights related to conflicts in a practice. If the conflict involves another area such as a financial or legal issue, you may look for a mentor who is experienced in that field. Remember that the mentor is only offering advice, and try not to use it in an inappropriate way toward the other party when trying to resolve the conflict. Additional information could also be obtained from other resources such as books, professional associations and trade magazines, and the Internet.

DISCUSS SOLUTIONS WITH ALL PARTIES INVOLVED

Set a time and place to meet with others involved in the conflict. Be sure to allow plenty of time for the meeting. A minimum of 45 minutes to an hour is usually needed. If only a few minutes were allowed, the conflict may not be resolved and the parties would likely walk away frustrated. It may be a good idea to hold the meeting outside the office. Choose a comfortable, relaxed location to set the mood for a more relaxed conversation. The choice of a public or private place may depend on the subject matter to be discussed. If private or confidential information is going to be discussed, a private location is better.

One of the parties may become emotional during the meeting. If one or more parties are angry, it may be appropriate to let them vent about what they feel has happened or why they are frustrated. It is also important to let everyone involved speak on the matter. Encourage others to go through the same process you already have and identify the problem, consider the facts, and consider all solutions and outcomes. You have done your homework, and it is important to allow the other person(s) involved to also go through these same steps. Often while going through this process, one of the parties realizes that its perception of the problem or the facts is inaccurate or limited. This is a good time to clarify the situation and a good step working toward a resolution. This is a good time to clarify the situation and can be an important step in working towards resolving a problem.

Talking about possible solutions and outcomes with all of the parties involved is a good way to validate that everyone is part of the process. If only one party makes decisions, generally others feel frustrated and left out of the process of resolving the problem.

COMPROMISE AND RESOLVE

Compromising in a small or large way allows everyone to seek a solution that will work for all. Being part of this process helps all parties make a conscious decision about what they can find acceptable (Fig. 12-5).

Once a resolution has been chosen, it is important to restate the decision. It may be a good idea to write down the decision to ensure that everyone comprehends the decision in the same way. This is also a good time for all parties to agree that, if the resolution does not work for them, they will meet again to work on another solution. Sometimes something new has to be tried before everyone knows how well it works. Leave the lines of communication open.

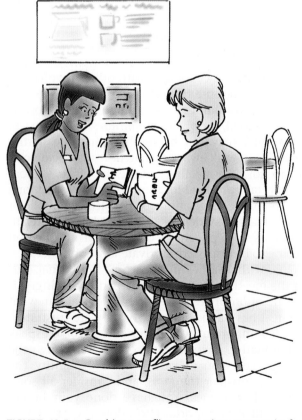

FIGURE 12-5 ■ Resolving a conflict may require a compromise from both parties.

CASE STUDY

Arlington Massage Works opened its office 2 years ago with five therapists who all graduated from the same massage school. All the therapists decided to develop their skills in different areas of massage and bodywork so they would not be competing against each other. Cynthia initially decided to become certified in NMT (neuromuscular technique) and Emily moved toward MFR (myofascial release) work. Cynthia later thought that combining NMT and MFR would help her clients get better results and took some classes in MFR. When Emily learned about this, she complained at an office meeting that they had all agreed not to compete against each other and now Cynthia was doing the same type of work that she was. She felt this would hurt her business and take away referrals from some of the doctors in town. Cynthia pointed out that she was seeking further education to help her clients and build her business. She felt that they all should accept learning new modalities and accept that sometimes therapies would overlap another's practice. She also pointed out that although they had orally agreed to this in principle when they opened the office, there was nothing stated in their written office policies about this issue. She apologized for creating a problem but felt that everyone in the office needed to think about this issue as it would probably come up again.

The five therapists each decided to write down areas that they wanted to train further in and bring their lists to the next meeting. They also decided to write down problems that might result from this cross-over and some solutions that could be sought.

The office found that working toward a positive resolution would keep the client focus of massage in the forefront of their work.

ETHICAL CONFLICTS

Sometimes a conflict situation involves an ethical conflict. While conflicts involving policies and procedures generally can be discussed in more objective terms, the ethics involved in a conflict may be more subjective and depend on a person's own beliefs. The ethical standards embraced by associations or groups are usually fairly well defined, but often there is room within these ethical standards for individual interpretations that may vary from person to person. In such cases, an existing policy may not necessarily resolve a conflict with an ethical solution. For example, if a facility does not require much draping, and in this state no laws regulate this aspect of massage, a therapist may have a personal belief or ethical standard that more draping should be provided for the client. Another example is a facility that does not use a health history form, but a therapist believes it is an ethical requirement to know about a client's health before performing a massage. The facility's schedule, however, may not allow enough time to do an intake interview. Here again, following the steps for conflict resolution can help solve this problem. Both parties should consider what is needed to ensure the client's well-being while still working within business parameters and the schedule.

Ethical solutions should not involve compromising ethical principles. The conflict resolution process should never contradict ethical or legal guidelines at the national, state, or local level.

EXERCISE 12-1

With a group of three or four students, take one of the cases listed below and, using the "Steps to Resolve Conflict," develop a solution for the problem. Each group should choose one person to write down the steps and associated actions. Then each group presents its case to the class, which can offer other possible solutions or compromises.

Case 1. Five therapists are practicing together. One therapist's friends frequently stop by the office and just hang out. Clients have mentioned these friends to the other therapists because they take up most of the space in the waiting room and often talk in unacceptable ways about massage. When this was mentioned to the therapist, he just laughed it off. What do you do?

Case 2. An employer receives a complaint from a client that her therapist had exposed her chest area during her massage. The client felt she had to hold onto the sheet to avoid further exposure. The client told the employer that when she said something to the therapist, the therapist seemed unconcerned. What should the employer do?

Case 3. Three therapists practice in an office together. One therapist decides to sell supplements and displays them in the waiting area without first discussing it with the other two therapists. Clients are now asking them about the supplements. What should the two therapists do?

Case 4. A client has received four sessions of bodywork for a work injury. The client was referred by a physician who requested only four sessions. The client tells the therapist that he is sure they can talk the doctor into more sessions, if the therapist would just say so. What should the therapist do?

SUMMARY

Conflicts are common in businesses that provide services for the public. Clients may find that they are unhappy with a service. More frequently, conflicts happen between employees, independent contractors, and employers. Policies and procedures can help prevent conflicts, but many areas are subjective in nature. Conflicts occur because expectations between two parties are not clear or communicated. It is important to resolve conflicts quickly so a therapist can concentrate on clients and their well-being. A practice that maintains ethical relationships with clients, other therapists, employers, employees, and other health care providers can focus more effectively on bodywork and massage.

SECRETS OF SUCCESS

- Importance of learning about ethics
- Ethical behavior as one of the key elements of success
- Making ethical behavior part of who you are
- Explanations by successful therapists of how ethics are important in their profession and in their lives

Ethical behavior has become one of the most frequently discussed subjects in the massage and bodywork community, along with the question of appropriate education for therapists entering this exciting profession. Students just enrolling in a massage therapy program typically do not think much about the role ethics will soon play in their lives and profession. Yet many educators have been talking for years about the importance of ethical behavior and the need for new students to understand and grow in this diverse and sometimes controversial area. In this chapter you will explore the journey that you have made thus far in this book in preparation for, in the last chapter, developing your own code of ethics for living and practicing in your new career. In this chapter successful therapists from the massage profession also offer their advice based on the influence of ethics on their careers.

SUCCESS IN THE MASSAGE AND BODYWORK PROFESSION

Many therapists and students are awed by individuals who seem always to do the right thing, whose schedules are full with satisfied clients, and who love their work. Many massage and bodywork professionals make a very good living, are happy with the work and services they provide for their clients, and are truly successful in their careers. On the opposite side, some other therapists train in bodywork, start to develop their career, falter, and then leave the profession, disappointed that they seemingly could not be successful in the massage field. It is important to understand why some individuals are successful while some are not.

KEY ELEMENTS OF SUCCESS

Three characteristics have a major role in determining a massage therapist's success:

1. Mind-set
2. Connection
3. Focus

The first important key to success is one's *mind-set.* The frame of mind of a new therapist entering the profession is important. Wanting to help others, having compassion, and being nurturing are important keys. Someone who enters this field motivated solely by the thought of making $60 or $70 an hour will likely be disappointed. As you will discover, much of that $70 an hour goes to overhead, purchases of supplies and equipment, and the advertising needed to start a business. As well, a therapist will not make $70 every hour of the day. For example, if you are working from 9 to 6, or 9 hours a day, you most likely give only five or six massages during that time. Most therapists schedule time to take a break or change over the room between clients.

The mind-set of a successful therapist goes beyond just wanting to help people while making a living. Successful therapists also enjoy the challenge of working with clients who need assistance to regain and maintain their health.

Simply performing a good massage is not enough. Understanding the dynamics of the human body, knowing how to work with those dynamics, and educating clients about physical changes are key elements of successful bodywork. Each massage client is unique and presents new challenges that the therapist and client confront together as a team. Even though massage therapy is a service industry, this teamwork approach must involve clients in the healing process. Clients want to understand why they have pain and do not always feel good. Explaining these matters and educating clients helps them be part of the process and connects the therapist and client in a unique one-to-one relationship.

A therapist's mind-set embracing professional ethics is also crucial for the client's safety and well-being. A client should never have to question a therapist's ethical foundation. As a student entering the field of bodywork and massage, you need to think about the ethical image you portray to clients. As you gain experience in the field, this mind-set will become second nature and part of who you are.

Connection with clients is the second key element in a successful practice. The first connection may begin on the telephone when a client makes an appointment or in person when the client first enters your office to receive a massage. When you first meet a client, during the first few moments the connection between the two of you is already developing. When two strangers meet the first time, they may instantly feel comfortable with each other or either or both may put their guard up. Clients are aware of how comfortable they feel with you during the intake interview. Their comfort level is affected even by your body language and the office atmosphere. The first few minutes with a client is a crucial time that strongly influences the development of the client–therapist relationship.

Therapists should make eye contact immediately with a client, shake the client's hand, and introduce themselves. A client who is filling out an intake form should be left alone for a reasonable time because having someone watching over you while filling out personal information can be intimidating. Clients are also likely to be more thorough when not feeling rushed. The intake interview should be done in a comfortable, quiet setting where you can truly focus on what the client is saying. Ask open-ended questions to learn more about what the client has written. An open-ended question is one that enables the client to give you more than just a yes or no answer. For example, therapists can ask clients to tell them about their headaches rather than asking if their headaches were caused by stress. The open-ended

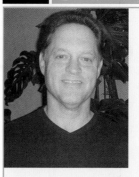

| BOX 13-1 | *Secrets for Success: Fred Engel, Springfield, MO* |

Here is a summary of my mind-set for my business from its inception: Integrity is everything. I don't want to be just like every other therapist in town. I want to be the one the other therapists call for treatment. When someone walks through my door looking for hope, I must do everything in my power to fulfill that need. I don't have any special powers. I'm just a regular person who facilitates the body's natural healing process. Advanced schooling is not an option—it is an absolute necessity. I must continually force myself out of my comfort zone. My very best marketing tools are my hands. The more often they are helping someone, the better the chances for referrals. Let every person know they are important. I listen with my heart. There is no room for jealousy. I try to motivate others to be successful by my example. Be professional, but make my clients feel comfortable. Be passionate about my profession. Let my clients know that I really do appreciate them. Know that I'm not going to be able to meet everyone's expectations. Spend quality time with my family and friends.

BIO

Fred Engel has been an entrepreneur for more than 20 years, with three other successful businesses in his past. He started his massage therapy business at the age of 52 and went into full-time practice in 6 months. His goal now is to expand his business to include wellness and nutrition.

question encourages clients to talk about how bad their headaches are or the location or frequency. If a therapist needs more information, he or she can then ask specific questions. A closed question, in contrast, usually elicits only a yes or no answer.

Jot down quick notes, which you can expand upon later after the session. Ask clients if they have any questions or concerns. You should be totally focused on the client's health and needs during the intake interview. Otherwise, the client will begin to feel a disconnect, which can begin even during the interview and then may set the stage for the rest of the session. A therapist who is interested only in doing the massage and not paying attention to the needs of the client will begin to alienate the client even during the initial interview. Clients expect a therapist to listen and connect with what they want to achieve from the massage session. It is not ethical for therapists to project their own thoughts or feelings for what a client should receive during a session.

Mr. Roberts was a frequent client at the massage therapy clinic in a training school. Students spent 6 weeks at the end of their program working in the clinic, and each performed at least 50 massages. Mr. Roberts was an honest client and often told the clinical supervisor what he thought of the student's work.

This week he received a massage from a female student who generally preferred to perform light work. Mr. Roberts liked heavier work, and the clinical supervisor wanted this student to get some practice in heavier work. This student was resistant to heavier work but did the massage.

After the massage, Mr. Roberts told the clinical supervisor that he did not like the massage. He said the student seemed really disconnected and just went through the motions. She never asked what he felt about the pressure, and whenever he told her he wanted deeper work in an area, she would get a bit heavier for just a minute or two and then go back to lighter work. He requested other students for his massages in the future.

When the clinical supervisor talked with the student about Mr. Roberts requesting other students in the future, she said she thought it didn't really matter since she probably would not be working on him again. The clinical supervisor told her that therapists are often challenged in the work they do. There is no such thing as a generic client. All clients come to their appointments with their own expectations, and if the massage does not meet their expectation, or their needs are not being met, they probably would not return. Connecting with clients involves talking with them about their expectations and working throughout the session to meet their expectations while educating them during the process.

Connecting with a client takes work. It is a continuous process that therapists should always be thinking about. Pay attention to both verbal and physical feedback from the client. If a therapist mentally disconnects from a client, the client will consciously or subconsciously feel it. The client may think, and may tell others, thoughts such as "The therapist didn't seem with it today" or "I don't feel like the therapist was paying attention to me or my needs." These are important comments. They show the client felt disconnected from the therapist and the client's needs were not met. Some clients may not consciously feel this but will leave the massage not sure why they did not like it, just knowing something was not quite right, and they will probably not return. The main goal of all client sessions should be to meet the client's needs, requiring the therapist to stay focused on the client.

To stay connected, therapists should constantly process the client's physical feedback and answers to the therapist's questions about the client's comfort or the area being worked on. Clients will understand the value of the therapist checking with them once in a while for some feedback. When a client comes for frequent sessions, it becomes easier to obtain feedback because the client usually feels more comfortable talking about things such as asking for lighter or heavier pressure. In addition, you can better interpret physical feedback, knowing how the client usually reacts.

A therapist can also become disconnected from a client by not listening to what the client is saying or not respecting the client's wishes. A therapist may do one type of work even though the client requested something else. If you feel a client would be better served by another type of work, discuss this with the client before beginning the session. For example, if a client wanted a deep tissue massage and the therapist failed to discuss this but performed only lighter work, the client will be disappointed. It is important that the therapist and client agree on the work to be done and the goal for the session before the work begins. Each client and each session can be uniquely different. It is unethical to perform work that a client is not expecting to receive. Educating each client about the work being done is an important component of bodywork.

Countertransference can also cause a therapist to disconnect from a client. Issues may begin to surface if the therapist begins to transfer thoughts and emotions to a client. As discussed in an earlier chapter, it is important for therapists to recognize the signs that this may be happening and to work to resolve the matter. A client should never be the target for a therapist's personal issues. Countertransference can cause significant disconnection, especially when a negative emotion is transferred.

Staying connected with clients takes practice and patience. Initially, new therapists are often more concerned with their techniques, pressure, body mechanics, and office issues. It can be challenging to keep the connection strong with each client or patient.

The third key element is *focus*. The mind-set and connection that therapists have with clients require focus. Clients expect the therapist to focus on them during a session. Clients generally do not want to hear about problems the therapist is having or the therapist's personal life. What clients do want to hear is information related to their condition or techniques that could be helpful for them.

Most clients are genuinely concerned about feeling better, and some are concerned about getting their money's worth from a session. Massage is not inexpensive, and many clients have to budget for an hour of massage or bodywork. A client who comes in with the expectation of feeling great after a stress-free hour will not be happy with a therapist who complains about his or her own problems during the client's time. It would not be ethical to charge a client to listen to your personal problems during their massage session.

Massage is considered a service profession. During the client's scheduled session, the therapist should set aside everything else and focus on the client. In the initial few minutes, explore the client's complaints and preferences and learn the client's goals for the session. Discussing options to help a client reach these goals helps the client see that you are seeking further information in order to best meet the client's needs. Restating in your own words what the client has said about his or her goals helps ensure that you both have the same thing in mind.

After you have escorted the client to the treatment room, you will have a few moments to collect your thoughts and plan what you will be doing during the session. You may think out a general plan, leaving room for some flexibility during the session as you physically connect with the client and let your intuition play a part in the treatment. Just before entering the room, take a moment to bring your awareness and focus to the client and let go of everything else related to your personal life and the business. During the session, if you feel your thoughts are beginning to stray, take a deep breath and bring the focus back to the client.

At times clients can distract the therapist from the massage. Some clients talk during a session out of nervousness, while others may simply be curious about the treatment or just like to talk. Many therapists say that it can be hard to focus when the client keeps asking questions. It is much like having two trains of thought at the same time: neither is given complete attention. Therapists report that they can even forget what body areas they have and have not worked on.

Box 13-3 describes some of the many subtle ways you bring the focus back to the treatment and get the feedback necessary for performing good bodywork.

When a client seems insistent on having a conversation, it may be best to stop the bodywork for a few moments and answer the client's questions. This lets clients know that you want to answer their questions but that your focus is lost on the work you are doing. When you are ready to return to the bodywork, suggest that the client focus on

---

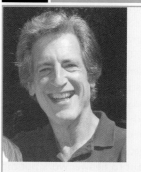

BOX 13-2 | *Secrets for Success: Elliot Greene, Silver Spring, MD*

One of the most compelling questions researchers have asked about the therapeutic process is what makes it work? What is the key to success? Investigating this question while preparing my book *The Psychology of the Body*, I found that research studies done by a number of the helping professions show that the single most powerful predictor of therapeutic outcome is the quality of the therapeutic relationship. I have also found this to be true in my own experience as a therapist. My ability to connect with my clients can be as important as—sometimes even more important than—the technique or method used. Furthermore, the more often a client comes for sessions, the more this comes into play. Therefore, it stands to reason that massage therapists need to focus on this aspect of their work as much as they do on acquiring and sharpening their hands-on techniques. The same is true, I would add, about massage therapy training.

Indeed, ethics and the therapeutic relationship are deeply linked. The purpose of ethics in massage therapy is commonly thought primarily to protect the interests and well-being of the client. However, ethics is more than a list of rights and wrongs. Upon digging deeper, one could say that much of the ethical framework is designed to protect and preserve the therapeutic relationship.

BIO

Elliot Greene, MA, NCTMB, has been a massage therapist for more than 33 years. He is the co-author of the book *The Psychology of the Body*; Lippincott, Williams and Wilkins; Baltimore, MD; 2004. Which explores the intricate connections between the mind and body and the underlying psychological factors and issues that influence the massage therapist–client relationship and the outcome of the therapeutic encounter. He is currently the president of the U.S. Association for Body Psychotherapy and a past national president of the American Massage Therapy Association (AMTA). He has received numerous awards honoring his contributions to the massage therapy field, including the AMTA Distinguished Service award, AMTA President's award, NCBTMB Founders award, and Massage Therapy Foundation Founders award.

---

the area where you are working and concentrate on relaxing that part. If all else fails, you may need to say something like this: "It is hard for me to focus on what I am doing if I'm talking. Can I answer your questions in a few minutes?" This lets the client know that you truly want to focus on the work and yet still want to answer the client's questions. Clients are generally not offended by such suggestions.

■ Before the session begins, tell the clients it is their time and they simply need to relax. Let clients know that you will be checking with them for comfort levels, but they should feel free to let you know what they are feeling about the pressure and how comfortable they are.

■ If a client seems nervous, beginning each new part of the body with very simple touch such as gentle rocking and soothing strokes can help the client to relax.

■ If clients start talking too much, ask them to focus on the part of the body you are working on. Ask them to try to help the area to relax by focusing on that part of the body and taking slow deep breaths to relax.

■ Ask clients to take some deep cleansing breaths. You may actually have to breathe in and out with them to help slow down their breathing.

■ During the breath work, suggest that clients try to let that part of the body go and relax into the table.

■ Ask clients to visualize their favorite place, such as the beach or a cool meadow.

WHY THERAPISTS ARE SUCCESSFUL

Massage therapists and bodyworkers are successful when they know the expectations of their clients and work to meet those needs. Bodyworkers frequently receive work themselves, and as consumers they know what they expect when they receive bodywork. Those expectations are not much different from those of the general public who receive massage.

After doing Exercise 13-1, you will likely see that most or even all students have very similar expectations. Paying attention to the client's expectations is one of the key elements to success. Throughout this chapter, successful therapists offer some of

EXERCISE 13-1

Write down five words that describe what you expect when you receive a massage or bodywork.

1. _____

2. _____

3. _____

4. _____

5. _____

Group discussion: After all the members of the class tell their five words and these are written on the board, the class then discusses similarities and differences among the answers.

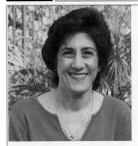

FOCUS AND INTENTION

Your session with your client is generally more successful and rewarding when you both are focused and your intentions are clear. You should ask your clients what they would like to take away from the session (state their intention) or what their expectations are. Then, establish and state how you plan to meet their expectations during the session (state your intention). At that time, both therapist and client should focus on what has been established as the goal.

For instance, if the clients' expectation is to feel more relaxed after the session, they can focus on a calm environment while you provide that calm environment through the atmosphere you provide and your touch.

Determining expectations, setting goals, and naming intentions helps assure a satisfying experience for both the therapist and the client. This leads to repeat bookings, client references, and increased business.

BIO

Chris Voltarel has more than 1,000 hours of massage education, in addition to her BA in Business Administration. She has been in practice since 1993 and an AMTA member since 1995. She has served in many volunteer positions with the AMTA, including Chapter President of the California Chapter and currently as Chair of the National AMTA Chapter Relations Committee.

their secrets about what they do and why it works. Massage techniques are very important, but having good hands is only one of the key ingredients for being successful.

Here's an important question to help you understand how important are the keys we have been discussing: If you were paying $75 for an hour of massage, what would you expect? Technique, skill, sanitation, and professionalism are all important, but focus, connection, and mind-set should be foremost. Take note, in the following sections, of what other professionals say are the important keys to their success.

> **Key Points**
>
> ■ Each client is unique and presents a new challenge for the therapist.
> ■ Clients will feel or not feel connected to the therapist.
> ■ Clients expect a therapist to focus only on them during their bodywork session.

ETHICS AND SUCCESS

Have you ever heard of an unethical massage therapist being successful? Most would define success in the bodywork profession as having clients who receive quality services and regain their health. Can you deliver quality services while being unethical? This is a very subjective question, and some may try to argue that quality services can be provided while being unethical. But more importantly, would you want to do this?

While in school, students learn a great deal about anatomy, techniques, pathologies, and applications. While all of these are important, so is ethics. A therapist who acts unethically will not keep clients even if he or she has excellent skills. For example, if a therapist performs great sports massage but gets new clients by telling people lies about other therapists, is this behavior ethical even in a world of cutthroat competition? Although a person may seem to get away with such behavior for a time, many believe such behavior will turn back on the person, and eventually this person will not be successful. The knowledge therapists need also includes understanding the importance of ethics and ethical behavior for a successful practice.

Knowing right and wrong is part of the self-exploration therapists should do throughout their training. Clients need to know that they can trust the therapist who is providing their treatment. Clients want to know that they do not need to worry about improprieties that could affect their session negatively. For example, if a client heard that his or her therapist had been accused of inappropriate behavior with another client, wouldn't this client think twice about returning to that therapist?

ETHICAL BEHAVIOR

Ethical behavior for bodyworkers means that the professional knows what is right and wrong when working with clients. Clients expect professionals always to treat them properly, even though some clients may purposely or inadvertently challenge a therapist. Opinions may sometimes vary, however, about what exactly is appropriate in certain circumstances. For example, one client may feel that it is right to expect a full hour treatment even if the client is 15 minutes late for the appointment. The client may feel that this is justified by paying full price for the session. The ethical argument on the other side, however, is that it is not appropriate to make the therapist late for other clients the rest of the day just because one client was late. Different people will naturally have differences of opinion on some aspects of ethics and behavior. Remember

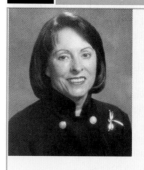

BOX 13-5 *Secrets for Success: Carolyn Talley-Porter, Greenville, SC*

Having worked in an orthopedic office for thirty years, I learned that ethics are not only important but are expected. I have been a massage therapist since 1992, when I began my business based on ethics and professionalism. Living in South Carolina, an area sometimes considered in "the Bible belt," we were already dealing with the old connotation of "massage parlors." The goals I set for my business were based on high standards, ethics, and professionalism. Ethical conduct has been important for my business as a massage therapist as well as teaching it as an instructor in our community college. Most all of my clients were referred to me because of my high standards of ethical practice and conduct. Because of this, my practice grew and became highly successful.

The public needs to feel safe and secure while receiving a massage from someone who is ethical and professional. I can't imagine a business surviving without these two characteristics.

BIO

Carolyn Talley-Porter's educational background is in business administration and management. She was an administrator for an orthopedic sports medicine clinic for 25 years. She attended the Fuller School of Massage in Virginia Beach from 1992 to 1994. Carolyn spearheaded legislation in South Carolina, which passed in 1996. She has been an active member of the AMTA, serving at the state and national levels, including National President from 2001 to 2002. She has been a volunteer with the AMTA Research Foundation helping to raise funds. Carolyn implemented the Massage Therapy Program at the Greer Campus of the Greenville Technical College in 1997 and owns Greenville Myotherapeutic and Sport Massage in Greenville, SC.

too that individuals were raised with different beliefs and backgrounds and have different life experiences. Ethical issues will therefore likely always involve differences of opinion in the massage profession.

Certain aspects of ethics in the bodywork profession *are* fairly clear, however, such as the principles of having no sexual contact with clients and maintaining confidentiality. These are easy to understand, and violations can often be proved. Other ethical areas such as those involving referrals and scope of practice involve more subjective issues, and practicing professionals often have a variety of opinions.

In all cases, however, therapists should be aware that their behavior will be constantly judged and analyzed by others, including their present clients and the general public. The public includes individuals who may be thinking about receiving bodywork and who might be skeptical and need assurance that the therapist is knowledgeable, trustworthy, and ethical. Clients generally have already developed a therapeutic relationship with a therapist and may think about ethics only if they are treated in a way they feel is inappropriate. All therapists should keep in the forefront the proper treatment of clients.

MAKING ETHICAL BEHAVIOR PART OF WHO YOU ARE

Chapters thus far in this book have contained much information and many ideas for new therapists to think about as they enter practice. By thinking about how their practice can be perceived by clients and the public, new therapists are better equipped to start their new careers.

Ethics and ethical behavior can easily and should become part of who you are. Once you have taken ownership of a code of ethics, it will become part of your behavior and everyday activities. Many ethical principles and guidelines will soon seem common sense in your practice. For example, if a client comes to see you with an illness that contraindicates massage, you will immediately understand the importance of referring that client to another health care provider. Similarly, if someone asks for information about one of your clients, ethically you will know that you cannot give any information regarding a client to another person without the client's permission. Simply saying that this is against your policies or code of ethics will become second nature.

When beginning a career in bodywork, it is often a good idea to find a mentor from whom to seek advice and counsel when you have questions regarding ethics as well as about business practices, treatment plans, conditions, or techniques. Your mentor may have experienced the same situation you are facing and can be a resource for information. Picking a mentor with a good reputation and experience in the field is important for your career. The mentor could be someone you are working for or who has his or her own practice. Many therapists begin by working in a facility where other therapists also work. These others can also be a good source of information.

In a practice with others, you may also see some things that you do not like, such as ways clients are treated or even ethical violations. It can be challenging to observe unethical behavior by others

BOX 13-6 *Secrets for Success: Cheryl Siniakin, Pittsburgh, PA*

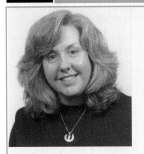

To me, ethics, which is derived from the ancient Greek word *ethos* meaning *character*, is not so much what I do as who I am, manifested in what I do. Ethics has been the cornerstone in my foundation as a human being as well as a massage therapist in private practice since 1977. "Doing the next right thing" is a principle that has directed, guided, and continues to build my character. I am continually personally evolving with the help and care of people who share their wisdom to help me foster my growth. I am constantly working with myself—emotionally, physically, and spiritually—to become more of who I am, and in that I find greater inner wisdom. In my own personal development, I strive to always be the student in my life and remain teachable, and to the best of my ability to know myself. My belief is that a key to my success as a massage therapist is knowing myself, as I have found that the clearer I am about who I am, the more available I am to help another.

One way that my character manifests in a massage therapy session is in deciding whether or not to work with a client. At the beginning of every appointment all clients shares with me their goals for the session. If I believe that they may benefit from the work I am able to offer, I work with them; and if I do not believe that my work can help them get to where they expressed wanting to go, I do not work with them. It is not my position to impose my sense of balance/health on my clients, but rather to accept them for who they are at each moment in time. Everyone has inner wisdom, and my clients do come to me for my skills, but that does not negate the inner wisdom that they possess.

"When 'do no evil' has been understood, then learn the harder, braver rule, 'Do good.'"

—Arthur Gutterman (1871–1943)

My clients appreciate the honor that I hold for their process. Each person has their own personal thumbprint in life. Magic happens during every massage session . . . and I am humbled and grateful to bear witness. Without a strong ethical foundation, none of this would be possible.

BIO

Cheryl L. Siniakin is a licensed Massage Therapy Instructor (LMTI) with a BS in Psychology and a PhD in Education and is Nationally Certified in Therapeutic Massage and Bodywork. Dr. Siniakin is National Bylaws Chair of the AMTA and past president of the Pennsylvania Chapter of the AMTA. Dr. Siniakin has been in private practice since 1977. She has trained and certified massage therapists since 1980. Dr. Siniakin is a certified Reiki Master, Reflexologist, and Bioenergetic Therapist. She is trained in On-Site Massage, Sports Massage, and Hypnotherapy. Dr. Siniakin is currently Associate Professor and Director of an Associate in Science Degree Program in Massage Therapy at the Community College of Allegheny County, Pittsburgh, PA. She is also the founder and director of the Pittsburgh Center for Health.

where you work. You may face a decision whether to say something to the manager or to move to another facility. It is important, in any case, not to give in to others' unethical behavior or let it affect your career and practice. Ethical behavior should become part of who you are, and staying committed to that behavior will help lead to a successful and safe career in massage.

> ### Key Points
>
> - Clients should expect to be treated ethically.
> - Therapists' behavior is judged by their clients and the public.
> - Working with a mentor will help with challenges and feedback.
> - Ethical behavior will become part of who you are.

BOX 13-7

Secrets for Success: Brenda Griffith, Richmond, VA

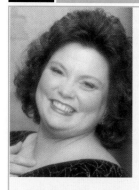

Your personal boundaries are one of the most important cornerstones for building your career as a professional massage therapist. Ethical boundaries have kept me grounded, and have allowed me to focus on building responsible professional relationships in all aspects of my career. Those areas include working with clients, association work with the AMTA, community education activities, teaching, mentoring, and local and state legislative projects.

Being true to your word and the commitments you make, keeping confidences, and being part of the solution and not the problem are all attributes derived from having a sound ethical foundation. When your ethical basis is firmly established, you have the tools to deal successfully with any situation you may face throughout your career; you will know what is acceptable and what is not, and you will be able to choose the correct course of action.

BIO

Brenda has been in private practice as a full-time massage therapist for 18 years. She has served at both the chapter and national levels of the AMTA since 1990 and was AMTA president from 2002 through 2004. Brenda volunteers as an on-site team member for the Commission for Massage Therapy Accreditation. She taught for 5 years at a local massage school and currently teaches continuing education courses on a limited basis.

WHAT SUCCESSFUL PEOPLE SAY

This chapter includes much insight from trained and experienced professionals in massage and bodywork. Most successful practitioners will tell you that ethical behavior is one of the key attributes of their success. Read carefully the words of the therapists in this chapter who have successful careers and offer their advice to you as a beginning therapist. These individuals have mentored many students and practitioners in this profession. Their success alone speaks highly for their ethical background and behavior.

SUMMARY

Ethics and ethical behavior are and should become part of who you are as a therapist. Throughout this text you have explored your own ethics and how your principles have developed, and you now clearly understand the importance of ethical behavior in your career. Successful therapists have shared insights that have helped them in their careers and that will help you realize the importance of ethics. Following your beliefs on what is right and wrong and building a strong ethical foundation will help you develop your own career.

ADDITIONAL ACTIVITIES

1. Make a list of contacts you may call upon when needing advice in the following areas:
   a. Business and legal issues
   b. Marketing
   c. Specific techniques that you wish to specialize in
   d. Psychological issues
   e. Support
2. List three resources besides a mentor to whom you can turn for information about ethics and standards of practice in the massage profession.
3. Write a paragraph about each of the following keys to success. List what you feel is important about each and some possible areas that you as an individual may need to work on or develop.
   a. Mind-set
   b. Connection
   c. Focus
4. List two ethical standards that you feel will be easy for you to follow. Then list two areas in which you feel you may still need some work. List actions that you can take to help you achieve those standards.

WRITING YOUR OWN CODE OF ETHICS

14

CHAPTER PREVIEW

- Understanding ethical issues by researching the ethical codes of other professions
- Gaining ownership of ethical behavior by writing your own code
- Need for thorough knowledge to achieve success in a profession

All individuals have their own personal code of behavior that they generally follow. Personal codes are generally unwritten and usually not communicated in full to others except when special needs arise. A code of ethics, in contrast, is a written document that a group, business, association, or individual presents to others, stating beliefs about appropriate and inappropriate behavior. Many massage and bodywork therapists belong to a group or association that has a code of ethics. When you join, you agree to follow that code. Some codes are written in general terms, while others may list very specific behaviors. In addition to these professional codes, all therapists should have their own personal code in order to feel personally safe and take ownership of what they do.

BUILDING ON EXISTING CODES

After reading previous chapters in this book, you should recognize the importance of having and following a code of ethics. Because published codes of ethics may seem too abstract or general, or may not feel personalized for your own beliefs and situation, it is a good idea to write your own code of ethics. Doing so gives you ownership of your code and your behavior in following it.

But it is not necessary to develop an ethical code entirely on your own—this would be a difficult and unnecessary endeavor. Many other massage therapists and other health care professionals have worked countless hours to develop the codes that exist today. Instead, building on those codes, you can develop a personal code of ethics that you can

call your own. The exercise in this chapter will help you clarify your beliefs, standards, and goals for your massage therapy practice. When you have completed your code, you can display it in your practice setting and include key parts in your marketing and advertising materials. Your code will help potential clients better understand your intentions as a therapist.

A personal code of ethics is a living document that you may change in the future as you see fit. Certain areas may be too rigid or confining, and others may need more definition or refinement. Every few years you should look closely at your code and decide if any changes are needed.

DEVELOPING YOUR OWN CODE

Writing your own code gives you, as a new therapist, a beginning foundation for your practice. It is challenging to begin a new career, but your code provides standards to which you can refer when needed. For example, if a client asks about another client, you can refer to a confidentiality standard that you have written. Exercise 14-1 requests that you include at least ten items in your code. This is a good number to start with, but feel free to expand your code to as many items as you feel are needed.

RESEARCHING PRACTICE ISSUES

Before you begin your practice, in addition to having a code of ethics, you should do some research to ensure that you have all the information you need affecting all areas of practice. This is true even

EXERCISE 14-1

Following the steps below, write your own code of ethics.

1. Read again the codes of ethics included earlier in this book and highlight or otherwise note statements in them that you like, feel comfortable with, and believe strongly in.

2. Look up other codes of ethics used by health care providers (psychologists, nurses, chiropractors, etc.) and highlight any parts that you feel are important. These ethical codes are commonly available on the Web sites of professional associations.

3. Write down any areas that are not included in these codes that you feel are important.

4. Go back through the items you have highlighted and write your own version of what you believe in. Carefully use your own words.

5. Write at least 10 individual items for your code.

6. Under each item in your code, write down two standards of practice for how you are going to achieve this item, in other words, an action step. For example:
   Code: Always protect the confidentiality of every client.
   Standards:
   a. Always keep client files in a secure, locked file.
   b. Never release a client's file without the client's signed permission.

7. Exchange your first draft of your code and standards with another student, and ask for suggestions for any changes in wording, punctuation, formatting, and so on.

8. Prepare a final document that you are comfortable sharing in your workplace. Your personal code of ethics can be displayed with other important documents in your practice and included in your brochure or advertising pieces.

CASE STUDY

Sandra was thrilled to find a location where she could begin to practice right after graduation from massage school. An established salon just a few miles from her house was looking for a massage therapist to work as an independent contractor in the salon. The salon needed someone right away because its former therapist had moved away and the salon had many requests for massages. Sandra had taken her national test and applied for her license as the state required. She felt ready to begin her practice.

Sandra was busy right away but soon felt uneasy about requests from some new clients. Several clients asked not to be draped. Because the previous therapist had not followed the state guidelines for draping, these clients felt Sandra should do the same thing. She spoke with the salon owner to see if this had previously had been an issue. He told her not to worry because no one would be checking. This did not make Sandra feel very comfortable because violating the draping guidelines could put her license in jeopardy and she did not feel it was ethical to do what the clients were asking. Sandra explained to her clients that she must follow the state guidelines.

A few weeks into her practice, the state inspector made a visit to the salon. He asked to see Sandra's license, which was in order, and also asked the salon owner to see his massage business license. The owner told the inspector that the massage therapist was practicing under his cosmetology license. The inspector informed them that this was not allowed and that he would have to apply for a massage therapy establishment license. The owner was not happy to learn about this regulation and decided he would not pay the $200 for the license. If Sandra wanted to continue to work there, she would have to pay this additional amount herself. Sandra then had to apply for and pay for the massage business license in order to continue to work at the salon. Sandra wished she had checked a little closer to make sure that all rules and regulations were being followed before she had started her practice.

if you are going to work for someone else in an established business. Unfortunately, some therapists have started practice and, only later on after having problems, learned about legal or ethical issues affecting them. Sandra's case is just one example of something that can happen to a new therapist starting practice without having thoroughly researched all practice and business issues.

Researching requirements for massage therapy practice is the responsibility of every therapist. It is not safe to rely on the word of a potential employer, who may not understand what is needed for a safe, ethical, and legal practice. In some cases a therapist may even have to educate a potential employer about meeting requirements to ensure that everyone avoids legal trouble. The research questionnaire included in Box 14-1 can help guide your research

| BOX 14-1 | *Research Questionnaire* |

LAWS AND ORDINANCES

1. What are the requirements in your state to practice as a massage therapist?

2. Do you need to take a test before applying for a state license?

3. What is the normal time period for testing and licensure? For example, the National Certification Exam application process usually takes about 4 weeks. You cannot apply until you have graduated and have the correct documents (transcript, diploma). Once you have been approved, you can set your test date within a 3-month period. You need to research the time needed to get the necessary documents from your school.

4. Is there a provision in your state law that allows you to practice while waiting to take the national test?

5. If the national test is required, once you pass the test, how long does it take to get the state license?

6. What local ordinances apply to a massage therapy practice? Check into ordinances such as home businesses, zoning, occupational licenses, and advertising.

7. Do you need to apply for a city or county business license?

PRACTICE ISSUES

Will you be working as an employee or independent contractor? (This is a very important issue when it comes to taxes and other issues affected by the delineation between a contractor and an employee. For more information, go to the IRS Web site and look under independent contractors.)

Independent Contractor

1. Will you be paying rent or working on a commission?

2. How often will you settle your accounts or be paid for your work?

3. Will you handle your own money or will someone else in the facility take care of it?

4. What expenses will you be responsible for (laundry, advertising, supplies, etc.)?

5. If discounts or specials are offered, who absorbs the cost?

6. Who books appointments? If it is someone else, who trains that person in the types of work offered, schedules, etc.?

7. What types of massage will be offered?

8. Who sets the schedule for therapists and session length?

9. In a business with multiple therapists, how are appointments handled? (For example, is there a rotating system if a client does not request a specific therapist?)

10. What company policies will apply to you?

Employee

1. Is the pay rate hourly or by session? Will you be paid during the times you are not performing massage?

2. How often will you be paid?

3. If discounts or specials are offered, who absorbs the costs?

4. Are there responsibilities other than massage? (For example, cleaning, laundry, receptionist, etc.)

5. Are you expected to assist in marketing, such as giving chair massages?

6. Who will be booking your appointments? If it is another person, who is responsible for training that person in what types of massage you offer and scheduling?

7. Working apparel: Are you required to wear a uniform and, if so, who pays for the clothing?

8. What types of massage or other treatments are you expected to do? If additional training is required, how is that done?

9. How long do the sessions last, and how much time is allowed between sessions?

10. What is the chain of command in the business? (For example, to whom should you go if a problem arises?)

11. If there are multiple therapists, how are the appointments handled if a client does not request a specific therapist? Is there a rotation system that makes it fair for all the therapists?

12. Do you have a copy of company policies?

13. Who pays for licensing or additional training?

before you invest time or money in a situation where problems could arise. For example, if a local ordinance states that a massage therapy business cannot be located in a certain area, you either have to look elsewhere for a location or work to have the ordinance changed.

Research your state and local laws and ordinances. Don't be afraid to go directly to sources such as state agencies or boards or local government offices; call these offices and ask for the information that you need. Obtain a copy of any ordinances

and laws that will apply to you. It is important that you obtain the information you base your practice on directly from the agencies or governments you will be dealing with. Obtaining information from other therapists or individuals can be dangerous because their information may be wrong or outdated.

RESOURCES

Without planning ahead, a new massage therapist could easily feel overwhelmed by the amount of paperwork and information needed to begin a practice. Yet it is not ethical to start a practice without the proper licensing and permits (Fig. 14-1). Many resources are available for therapists opening a business or working for someone else. One can easily be confused about what it means to practice as an independent contractor, for example. Researching IRS requirements will help you know the expectations for a therapist and business owner.

The Internet is a valuable resource, but don't be afraid also to go to your city hall or county office to ask for copies of ordinances or laws that apply to your massage therapy practice. In some states, a therapist is required to pass a test, apply for a state license as a massage therapist, apply for a state massage business license, and apply for a local city business license. It is important to know the requirements and plan for the

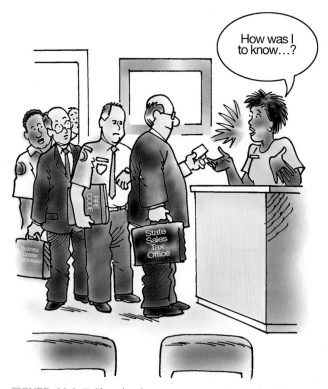

FIGURE 14-1 ■ Plan ahead to open your practice with all licensing in place and local conditions met.

time and expenses involved. Knowing the needed steps also helps you plan when and where to begin practice as a massage therapist.

SUMMARY

One step at a time, educate yourself on the requirements for practice in your area. Talking with a mentor or instructor who can help guide you will make these tasks easier. When all the proper documentation is in place and you understand what is required of you, you can begin your rewarding career as a massage therapist. Knowing that you did things the right way will give you confidence to begin your practice with a strong foundation and the information you need to be successful. Be proud of your accomplishments and always stand on your ethical foundation. It will serve you well. Congratulations on your new career!

GLOSSARY

Accountability: showing the responsibility or proof of performing a task or duty

Beliefs: what you personally feel is true

Boundaries: limits between acceptable and unacceptable behaviors

Civil law: system of law involving relationships or disputes between two parties

Code of ethics: a document stating an individual's or group's beliefs, standards, and ethical expectations

Conflict: a condition that occurs when two or more people have different attitudes or ideas about how something should be done or when a person has to choose between two inconsistent actions

Consultation: the process of obtaining advice from another professional in the same or related field

Countertransference: a therapist attributing thoughts or feelings about another person to the client

Criminal law: system of law regarding actions that are harmful to the public

Culture: the customary beliefs, habits, and traits of a racial, religious, or social group, often depending on one's country and language

Defense mechanisms: behaviors that unconsciously protect a person from feelings or awareness

Disclosure: revealing information to another person about oneself or another person.

Dual relationship: a situation that occurs when two roles or relationships overlap or interact

Emotional boundaries: limits for keeping therapeutic sessions focused on the client's body rather than on emotions

Ethics: an individual's or group's standards of behavior

Independent contractor: a non-employee who provides services within a business

Informed consent: a client's right to all pertinent information about a treatment and the granting of permission for a treatment based on that knowledge

Intake form: a form used in most practices in which clients provide information about their health, contact information, and other information that a therapist or other health care provider deems pertinent

Laws: rules established and enforced by governing bodies that protect or restrict actions by all citizens or specific parties

Morals: beliefs about what is right and wrong or good and bad

Ordinances: rules and regulations established at the local level

Physical boundaries: the physical lines or limitations in relation to a client's body that a therapist should not cross

Policies: rules and guidelines established for a particular group or population, such as a business

Power differential: the shift of authority that can exist in the client–therapist relationship

Procedures: processes by which policies and guidelines are carried out

Professional boundaries: the limits of acceptable professional behavior

Professional courtesy: a professional doing a favor for another professional

Professional ethics: a consensus of a group or association about its expectations concerning ethical principles and behavior

Referral: the process of sending a client to another professional for care

Regulations: rules of conduct that are often associated with laws, involving an expansion or explanation of the laws

Resolution: a solution found or formulated to end a conflict

Safety zone: the client's physical areas that a therapist may touch without provoking anxiety; also referred to as the client's "comfort zone"

Scope of practice: a definition or set of parameters for activities a professional is or is not allowed to perform as defined by the professional's competency, training, and/or laws and regulations

Self-regulation: process by which a group, association, or profession sets guidelines, expectations, and repercussions for inappropriate behavior

Sensuality: a feeling of pleasure gained from the stimulation of one or more of the senses

Sexual boundaries: limits to prevent ever sexualizing any aspect of bodywork

Sexuality: the emotional, physical, cultural, or spiritual actions or reactions related to sexual arousal

Social boundaries: limits for keeping the relationship with clients professional rather than social

Sole proprietor: a person who owns and operates his or her own business and often works alone

Standards of practice: accepted way in which ethical behavior is performed

Supervision: working under the direction of another professional

Third-party disclosure: giving information about a client to an outside person or entity

Transference: a client attributing thoughts or feelings about another person to the therapist

Values: something of worth or held in esteem

INDEX

Note: Page numbers followed by *f* refer to illustrations; page numbers followed by *t* refer to tables or boxes.